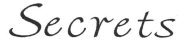

Secrets from a Healthy Asian Kitchen

OTHER BOOKS BY YING CHANG COMPESTINE

Cooking with Green Tea

Secrets of Fat-Free Chinese Cooking

The Runaway Rice Cake
(Simon and Schuster Books for Young Readers)

The Story of Chopsticks (Holiday House)

The Story of Noodles (Holiday House)

The Story of Kites (Holiday House)

The Story of Paper (Holiday House)

壽

Avery

A MEMBER OF
PENGUIN PUTNAM INC.
NEW YORK

Secrets from a Healthy Asian Kitchen

Ying Chang Compestine

5

641.595
COM

AVERY

a member of
Penguin Putnam Inc.
375 Hudson Street
New York, NY 10014
www.penguinputnam.com

Library of Congress Cataloging-in-Publication Data

Compestine, Ying Chang.
    Secrets from a healthy Asian kitchen / Ying Chang Compestine.
        p.   cm.
    Includes index.
    ISBN 1-58333-127-1
    1. Cookery, Asian.   I. Title.
    TX724.5.A1C64   2002   2001056647
    641.595—dc21

Printed in the United States of America

10   9   8   7   6   5   4   3   2   1

This book is printed on acid-free paper. ∞

Book design by Jennifer Ann Daddio

To China,

the country that

taught me how

to eat healthily.

ACKNOWLEDGMENTS

There is not one day when I don't feel blessed to be able to do what I like most: cook, eat, write, travel, and share my creations with others.

A special thank-you goes to publisher John Duff at Penguin Putnam for providing me with the opportunity to publish this book. Thank you for your confidence and trust in me.

Thanks to my dear friend and executive editor, Laura Shepherd, for your encouragement and professional guidance throughout this book. Thanks for showing your enthusiasm by testing my recipes on your friends and family. I'm so proud that people say you are a great cook when you serve my dishes.

Thanks to Dara Stewart, Avery editor, for your generous efforts in bringing this book to a higher state of excellence.

Thanks to my friends at *Cooking Light* magazine. You are the most talented and dedicated group I know. Thank you, Jill Melton, for your friendship throughout the years. I have learned so much by working with you.

I would also like to thank the following companies for providing their high-quality products for use in recipe development: KitchenAid, Ducane, Calphalon, Henckels, Zojirushi, and Eden Foods.

I want to use this opportunity to extend my thanks to the following friends for their enduring support and encouragement: Diane and Fred Glover, Valerie Crecco, Amy Gahran, Tom Vilot, and Roger Stevens.

Thanks to my son, Vinson, for telling me how much he missed my good food when I was away. It makes me feel irreplaceable and loved. Each day you add so much joy and happiness to my life!

And last but not least, to my husband, Greg, who continues to be my taste tester and my writing critic. You are the wind beneath my wings.

Contents

INTRODUCTION

Fifteen years after coming to America, at night I still dream of life in China. One frequent dream takes me back to when I shopped with my grandmother in the morning vegetable markets where we bought fresh vegetables, fruit, and spices for the family.

As a child I always enjoyed those shopping trips. Grandmother stopped often to chat with friends while I filled our basket with my favorite fruits and vegetables. On the way home, we stopped at the tofu stands to pick out different types of freshly made tofu. Often the steam would still be rising from the crisp, white blocks. For breakfast, Grandmother sometimes broke open the fresh tofu and drizzled in a little honey. I would devour the tofu along with a steamed bun and a cup of soymilk.

China surrounded me with the earth's abundance. I grew up in Wuhan, a city straddling the Yangtze River in south-central China. The river provides an ancient corridor for trade to the eastern and western provinces of China, while rail lines stretch to the north and south. At this crossroads, crops came to us from every point on the compass. In the spring we had mangoes, pears, papayas, watercress, mushrooms, and green beans from the south. Summer brought locally grown tomatoes, corn, cabbage, carrots, turnips, cucumbers, all varieties of peppers, and delightfully sweet watermelons. Giant apples arrived from the north in the fall, competing with juicy grapefruits from the east. Winter came with lotus roots, water chestnuts, black mushrooms, winter melon, and sugarcane from the south. I miss the clean breeze off the river, the colorful fruit, and the happy, friendly noises of the market.

In her kitchen, my grandmother prepared fresh vegetable and tofu dishes for us in many different ways every day. She seasoned various sauces with fresh chili pepper, garlic, ginger, and green tea. She soaked the sweet rice overnight, then ground it into dough. She used fresh fruit and sweet bean paste as fillings for delicious desserts.

For many years, we ate fully flavored food with complete enjoyment. While we were unaware that we were eating a nutritious diet, this food ensured that my brothers and I grew up healthy, and it taught us respect for nature.

As an adult, I have opportunities to travel all over Asia and other parts of the world. Each place I go I put a lot of time and effort into searching out the best food; I am fascinated with food. I strongly believe that food reflects the culture and customs of a country. After eating, I create recipes for my books.

The Secrets of a Healthy Asian Kitchen

Traditionally, the Asian diet has been purported to have health benefits, including preventing cancer and obesity. Unfortunately, as western culture and food is introduced, that is changing somewhat. Public health officials in Asian countries are growing alarmed by the changing diet in their populations. Major differences in eating habits are appearing between urban and rural people in the developing world. The diets of young people in cities have become more westernized, especially in large and medium-size cities. For a long time, Asian public health agencies were mainly concerned with the diseases of malnutrition that accompany scarcity and poverty. Now they have to deal with the fast-rising rates of the chronic diseases of affluence that accompany westernized diets rich in saturated fats. The number of cases of diabetes could triple if the dietary changes and obesity rates continue. Clearly, Asians were not protected from chronic diseases by any genetic advantage. Their advantage lies in their traditional Asian diet.

One thing I've learned about all Asian cooking is that it relies on fresh herbs, spices, and ingredients. All the dishes are not only aromatic but also well balanced. For thousands of years in Asia, food was for more than just sating hunger; it was also for maintaining good health. Research has shown that low rates of certain types of disease in Asia are due to the diet. Studies show garlic's ability to protect against stomach cancer and heart disease; ginger's ability to lower cholesterol; soy's ability to ease menopause symptoms; shiitake mushroom's antioxidant and anticancer benefits; ginseng's power as an immune system stimulant and its ability to improve both mental and physical performance; and green tea's ability to inhibit the production of carcinogens and promote weight loss.

THE ASIAN FOOD PYRAMID

The first secret of a healthy Asian kitchen is captured by the Asian Food Pyramid and its similarity to the U.S. Dietary Association (USDA) guidelines for healthy eating.

Scientists and researchers from such prestigious universities as Cornell, Harvard, and New York University have been studying the health effects of traditional Asian diets. Perhaps the most important result of this research is the Asian Food Pyramid. The nonprofit foundation Oldways Preservation and Exchange Trust, working in association with Cornell and Harvard University researchers, developed the official version of this pyramid.

The Asian Pyramid differs from the USDA pyramid in that it recommends that meat be eaten less often and in smaller amounts. Most of the daily protein comes from such vegetarian sources as legumes, seeds, and nuts. It emphasizes minimally processed foods, daily physical exercise, and consumption of the plant-based beverage tea.

The Asian Food Pyramid captures the healthy aspects of the traditional cuisine of the Pacific Rim, including the countries of Japan, Indonesia, Malaysia, the Philippines, India, Thailand, and China. The pyramid reflects

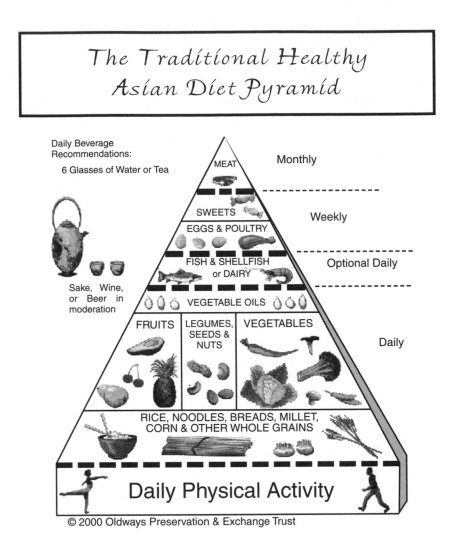

The Traditional Healthy Asian Diet Pyramid

Daily Beverage Recommendations:

6 Glasses of Water or Tea

MEAT — Monthly

SWEETS — Weekly

EGGS & POULTRY

FISH & SHELLFISH or DAIRY — Optional Daily

Sake, Wine, or Beer in moderation

VEGETABLE OILS

FRUITS | LEGUMES, SEEDS & NUTS | VEGETABLES — Daily

RICE, NOODLES, BREADS, MILLET, CORN & OTHER WHOLE GRAINS

Daily Physical Activity

© 2000 Oldways Preservation & Exchange Trust

the largely vegetarian diets of rural people. This diet has been associated with lower rates of certain cancers, heart disease, obesity, and in some cases, chronic, degenerative diseases such as osteoporosis.

"The Asian diet meets every recommendation you can think of for what you need to help prevent chronic disease," says Dr. Marion Nestle, Chairperson of the Department of Nutrition and Food Studies of New York University.

". . . the Asian diet, which is significantly lower in total fat, may prove to be an even more healthful diet," says T. Colin Campbell, Cornell professor of nutritional biochemistry. He is the cochair and director of the Cornell-China-Oxford project, which surveyed more than ten thousand families in mainland China and Taiwan to study diet, lifestyle, and disease.

Among their findings: Chinese people have half the cholesterol levels, lower cancer rates, much lower heart disease rates, and lower average body weight than their American counterparts.

For years, Americans have been told that dairy products will prevent osteoporosis. "Yet, the plant-based, dairy-free diets of much of Asia are linked to a low rate of osteoporosis," Campbell noted. "In fact, Western countries, with their calcium largely taken in the form of dairy products, have significantly higher rates of osteoporosis." Campbell said he hopes that the Asian Food Pyramid will bring further attention to the evidence that there are many traditional cuisines worldwide that are useful in promoting good health.

To my surprise, I found that the average Chinese consumes 20 percent more calories than the average American, yet Chinese cholesterol levels are lower. Why? Because only 15 percent of the calories come from fat, while in America up to 40 percent of the calories come from fat.

Americans also eat one-third more protein than the Chinese, and most of that comes from animals. Less than 7 percent of the Chinese diet is composed of animal protein. According to Dr. Campbell, a diet with excess protein, especially animal protein, may have the greatest potential for increasing the risk of the so-called diseases of affluence: cancer, heart disease, and diabetes.

THE CONCEPT OF YIN AND YANG

The second secret to a healthy Asian kitchen is founded in the wisdom followed by the Chinese for thousands of years. *Yin and yang* is a concept first formulated by Lao-tzu, the father of Taoism, who lived in the sixth century B.C. He taught his belief of opposites in balance to Taoist monks, who helped spread the concept throughout China. The term describes interrelationships within the circle of the universe. All life within it contains this pairing of

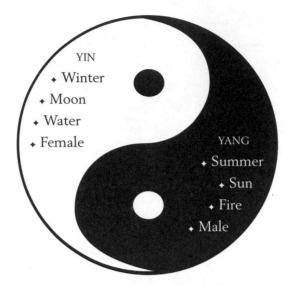

YIN
- Winter
- Moon
- Water
- Female

YANG
- Summer
- Sun
- Fire
- Male

opposites. They represent the opposing yet unifying forces of every action and object. Together they make up the whole circle. Yang is active and warm, while yin is passive and cool. Harmony occurs only when these two forces are in equal balance.

Based on traditional Chinese medicine, a healthy person is one with balanced yin (passive) and yang (active). The key concept of Chinese medicine is that sickness and disease are a result of an imbalance of yin and yang.

According to Lao-tzu, "To see the disease, first look at the diet." It is important to find balance in cooking and eating. Too much yin food will cause the body to produce only yin energy—slow movement, feeling chilled, and low energy. Too much yang food causes the body to produce only yang energy—fast, hot, and aggressive. During certain times of life and different seasons, a person may require more yin or yang food. For example, you may need yang foods to restore energy after an illness, or if you are a new mother recovering from birth, during cold weather, or after a long, hard workout.

Growing up with a mother who was a doctor of traditional Chinese herbal medicine, I learned at an early age about the importance of the pursuit of harmony. Mother frequently examined our tongues and pulses to measure our *qi*, which represents vital energy. She used yin and yang terms to describe the function and quality of our *qi*. Mother arranged our daily menu based on the season and our bodily condition. Many days our meals were decided after Mother's checkup. Mother believed that food plays a major role in our health. She explained to me later on that Chinese doctors divide food into three categories: hot, cold, and neutral (see the list below). Based on our individual yin and yang conditions, sometimes we were instructed to eat different types of food: cold (yin), hot (yang), or neutral (a balance of yin and yang).

COOLING FOODS	WARMING FOODS	NEUTRAL FOODS
Asparagus	Chili peppers	Broccoli
Bean sprouts	Chives	Green beans
Celery	Cilantro	Green onions
Chinese cabbage	Garlic	Oyster mushrooms
Crabmeat	Ginger	Shiitake mush-
Cucumber	Honey	rooms
Lemongrass	Leeks	Snow peas
Melon	Onions	Spinach
Mung beans	Orange	Sweet potatoes
Napa cabbage	Pumpkin	
Seafood	Red meat	
Squash	Toasted nuts	
Tofu		
Watercress		
Zucchini		

We were not allowed to consume too many yin foods in the wintertime, such as cold water, raw vegetables, or cold food. Instead we were served yang foods to increase the speed of digestion and metabolism. These included such foods as thick broth, food cooked with Chinese ginseng, and pungent spices such as chili pepper, ginger, and garlic. In the summertime we were served yin foods that were easy to digest and helped augment body fluids and slow down the metabolism, such as light soups, steamed rice, mushrooms, green vegetables, and tofu. Most meals were a harmonious balance of yin and yang adjusted for the seasons: green vegetables cooked with pungent spices, meat served with vegetables and steamed rice, and so forth.

After moving to America, during our phone conversations, I frequently received diet instructions from my mother. No ice cream in winter, avoid large amounts of red meat in summer. Eat a balanced, neutral diet by including grains that provide a good balance of yin and yang in every meal. Remember to balance and flavor the food with natural ingredients such as ginger, garlic, green tea, ginseng, and mushrooms. Avoid monosodium glutamate and excess sugar and salt.

Throughout this book you will find detailed information on healthy Asian ingredients, useful cooking tips, and colorful insights into the history and culture of Asia—even some Asian beauty secrets. The recipes contain healthy ingredients that people in Asia have used for thousands of years. Many are accompanied by a personal story, information on its health effects, the history behind the dish, or timesaving tips.

Vegetarians will find numerous recipes for their tastes—recipes that show just how easy it is to cook satisfying dishes without meat. Most of the recipes in this book are dairy-free. People sensitive to wheat will find many recipes without wheat-based products. In addition, rice and bean noodles can often replace wheat noodles. The traditional spring roll wrapper, made from wheat flour, can be replaced with a rice wrapper.

In recent years, the wholesome nature of the Asian diet has attracted a great deal of attention in America. More Asian ingredients and products are becoming available at the market every day. By combining readily available, nutritious products with modern kitchen equipment, you will discover how simple it is to make all these delicious dishes.

While you are enjoying the tasty food made from the recipes in this book, you will also be enhancing your health. Although the recipes have an Asian touch, I have modified them to fit American lifestyles and tastes. I have also included western recipes that use healthy Asian ingredients. These dishes reflect a wide range of East and West cuisines.

Whether you are a new cook or an experienced chef, you will find these recipes complete and easy to follow.

1. The Six Key Ingredients to a Healthy Asian Kitchen

In the Introduction, you read about the Asian Food Pyramid, which emphasizes a diet that is primarily plant-based. Of course, this is the main secret to a healthy Asian diet. But there are six particular ingredients that I have found to be the foundation of a healthy Asian kitchen. All of these ingredients have played a significant role in Asian cuisine and culture and are noted for their health-promoting properties by both traditional Asian medicine and modern western medical research. In this chapter, I will introduce you to those six key ingredients.

Ginger

My first memory of ginger is from the spicy-warm aroma of ginger candy. As a child, when I had a tummy ache or travel sickness on a long bus ride, Grandmother offered me a piece of ginger candy made from young preserved ginger rolled in fine sugar. When I had a cold, Grandmother was there with a cup of hot sweet ginger tea. My mother, a doctor of traditional Chinese herbal medicine, treated her patients with ginger for nausea, stomach problems, colds, joint pain, and frostbite. She called ginger "a gift from nature." As you might imagine, my memories of ginger are linked with sweet, warm, and caring feelings.

11

People throughout Asia have long valued ginger as a treasure of home remedies and culinary delights. The earliest record of ginger's medical use dates back five thousand years to the Chinese medical book *Manual of the Celestial Husbandman*. Doctors in China and India called ginger "the universal medicine."

The ginger plant—*Zingiber officinale* or *Zingiberis rhizoma*—is a member of the tropical family Zingiberaceae. It is thought to have originated in the tropical and subtropical regions of Asia. From there it spread to the rest of the world. Many believe that ginger may be one of the first plants cultivated by humankind.

Today ginger's uses extend far beyond our kitchens. Ginger extracts, ginger oil, and ginger essence are widely used in medicine, perfumes, beverages, and processed foods.

Ginger grows incredibly well in tropical and subtropical climates. A perennial, the ginger plant grows in shady places up to a meter in height. It has bamboolike stems and leaves. The greenish flower is sweetly perfumed. The skin of gingerroot is usually a shade of beige, although some varieties can have a lighter color, ranging even to a pale greenish white.

The color, aroma, and flavor of the gnarled gingerroot is affected by the soil and climate in which it is grown. The ginger we buy in the United States comes from Asia and Central America, and from Hawaii, which is famous for its young or "baby" ginger.

The root is often called the "hand," since it vaguely resembles a fat, gnarled hand. The root's skin is thick and flaky.

GINGER AND YOUR HEALTH

Asian medicine has employed ginger as a treatment for asthma, shortness of breath, water retention, earaches, diarrhea, nausea, and vomiting for thousands of years. Today homeopathic practitioners recommend it for sexual disorders as well. In the yin/yang concept of harmony and Chinese medicine, ginger is considered yang and warm. A study conducted by Professor Izrael Brekhman's team, from the Far East Science Center of the former Soviet Union, found that ginger was the fifth most frequently used remedy in the

Orient. It is believed to be able to warm the body, improve blood circulation, activate the body's defenses, and to relax the muscles of the stomach. It has also been found to help fight viral infections, including colds and flu; lower cholesterol levels; act as an anti-inflammatory agent and pain reliever, including in the treatment of arthritis and migraines; and aid digestion and assist the absorption of food.

Ginger contains many different substances that benefit our bodies. But scientists believe the two most effective ingredients are the pungent, fragrant ingredients *gingerol* and *shogaol*, which are key to ginger's therapeutic effects.

BUYING AND STORING GINGER

There is a wide variety of ginger products on the market. Ginger's flavor can range from very mild to a burn that takes your breath away and squeezes out the tears. Ginger is available in several forms.

Young "Baby" Ginger

Young fresh ginger has a creamy color with pink-tipped shoots. It is mildly flavored and has a wonderful, less fibrous texture. It is ideal to use for seafood and desserts. Its thin skin doesn't need to be peeled. Young ginger can be found in the health-food store. It is mostly available in early summer, and some health-food stores carry it year-round.

Old "Mature" Ginger

This is the fresh ginger that we usually see in the market. It has more fiber, is more fragrant and more strongly flavored than young ginger. Because of its strong nature, a little bit can go a long way. It is good for soups, stews, meat dishes, and some sauces.

BUYING FRESH GINGER

Even though we speak of fresh ginger, "fresh" is not really accurate. After the harvest, ginger is sun-dried for a short time to help it travel without spoiling. Look for ginger that is plump, firm, and not too fibrous. Avoid ginger hands with wrinkled skin or ones that feel light. When sliced, the fibrous flesh of the root ranges from pale to bright yellow. If the flesh has a bluish tinge to it, it's a sign that the ginger has begun to dry. I like "hands" with lots of fingers and knobs. This makes it convenient to cut off a chunk for the evening's meal. I believe that no other form of ginger can replace fresh ginger.

STORING FRESH GINGER

Fresh ginger will keep for several weeks if it's kept dry and cool. If you are going to use the ginger within a week, place it in a brown paper bag in your fruit bowl on the kitchen counter. You don't have to refrigerate it. For longer storage, first wrap it in a paper towel, then in a brown paper bag. Store it in your vegetable crisper in the refrigerator. It will last up to four weeks, as long as you make sure the paper towel is dry and absorbs moisture from the ginger. Or you can store the ginger like the Chinese do: bury it in your rice jar (see the instructions for how to store ginseng on page 32). In general, I don't like to freeze fresh gingerroot. It turns to mush when thawed.

POWDERED GINGER

Ginger powder is ground from dried, mature ginger. It is used in sweet preparations such as cookies, cakes, and puddings. It is best to buy small amounts of good-quality ground ginger, as the volatile essential oils that make up the flavor are easily lost to the air. Store in a tightly sealed container. It will last for several months.

PRESERVED GINGER

These young tender roots are harvested at about six months of age. They are cooked whole or in pieces and steeped in sugar syrup for a few days before being packed. Store in a sealed container in a cool, dry place. It will last for several months. I use preserved ginger in desserts. Preserved ginger can be found at your local Asian market or gourmet food store.

CRYSTALLIZED GINGER

After being preserved, the ginger is drained and rolled in fine sugar. It is sold as a candy and as an ingredient for the baking and confectionery industry.

Store in a sealed container in a cool, dry place. It will last for several months. You may be able to find crystallized ginger in the dried fruits and nuts section of your grocery store. Otherwise, it is sold at natural-foods stores and Asian markets.

PICKLED GINGER

Thinly sliced ginger is preserved in vinegar. The best-known type is sushi ginger, which is pickled in rice vinegar. Check the expiration date on the bottle before purchasing and store in the refrigerator. You can buy pickled ginger from an Asian market or health-food store.

PREPARING AND COOKING WITH GINGER

For sauce and fillings use minced or grated ginger to get the most flavor. For fast-cooking dishes, such as a stir-fry, cut ginger in small pieces or shred it. Use bigger chunks of ginger for dishes that require a longer cooking time, such as stews and soups. Use young ginger for mild sauces, seafood, and desserts and mature ginger for strong sauces, meat, and main dishes.

It is not necessary to peel young ginger, but it's best to peel mature ginger. A simple, quick way to peel ginger is to use a spoon or a small knife. Sometimes I simply cut it into big, easy-to-handle chunks. I place the chunks on a cutting board, flat side down, and shave off the skin with a sharp knife. Once they are peeled, I shred or mince the chunks.

Although the amount of ginger in one recipe is not enough to have a medicinal effect, remember the old Chinese saying, "Build a strong house with good bricks." As with other medicinal foods, ginger has long-term preventive health benefits.

At an early age, I learned to value ginger as a treasure of culinary delights and home remedies. Ginger is an ideal hot ingredient that complements yin ingredients such as vegetables, seafood, white meats, and fruit. Because the pungent taste of ginger is full of fire and warmth, it is the best ingredient for balancing cooling foods and enhancing a delicious dish.

As impressive as ginger's health benefits are, it can have an even bigger impact on our food. I couldn't imagine cooking a meal without ginger. I include it in soups, desserts, and everything in between. I use it with fresh vegetable dishes to balance the yin and bring out their fresh flavor. I use it to remove "fishy" odors and bring out the fresh taste of seafood. Ginger counteracts any gaminess in red meats, enhances flavors in poultry dishes, and helps tenderize meats.

Garlic

Interestingly, garlic's history reaches back to two of our oldest civilizations: Egypt and China. We know that garlic was fed to the laborers that built the pyramids of Giza, and that garlic was used in embalming by the Egyptians. It was also an important part of the diet of soldiers in ancient Rome.

Chinese scholars wrote about garlic as early as 3000 B.C. Chinese medicine considers garlic a yang or warm food.

Garlic has been cultivated for so long that it now depends on people for its reproduction. Garlic plants rarely produce seeds, so crops are grown from the cloves of a previous harvest. It's a wonderful plant for the garden. Many hardy varieties are available. Some need to be exposed to the cold for proper growth; plant in the late fall or very early spring.

GARLIC AND YOUR HEALTH

If you think garlic is just for seasoning, think again. Garlic contains hundreds of compounds. Researchers believe that *allicin* is the most important of these as a contributor to garlic's health effects.

Louis Pasteur noted in 1858 that bacteria died when they were doused with garlic. At the turn of the century, garlic was the drug of choice for tuberculosis. Albert Schweitzer used garlic to treat cholera and typhus. And during World War II, British physicians treated battle wounds with garlic. In Russia, it's called Russian penicillin.

Cholesterol Reducer

In more than two hundred studies of people with high cholesterol, one-half to one whole garlic clove a day typically lowered their levels by about 9 percent. Benefits showed up in a month, and also came from garlic supplements. Tufts University's *Diet and Nutrition Letter* suggests two cloves of garlic a day might be as potent as some cholesterol-lowering drugs.

Artery Protector

A newly discovered garlic plus: It prevents the bad cholesterol (LDL) from oxidizing, a process that initiates plaque buildup on artery walls, which can lead to clogging, heart attack, and stroke. The theory is that unoxidized cholesterol is not very harmful. So garlic eaters might have less harmful cholesterol than nongarlic eaters with identical cholesterol counts.

Blood Thinner

Studies suggest that garlic compounds help thin the blood, says Eric Block, professor of chemistry at the State University of New York at Albany. Block has isolated a garlic chemical, *ajoene* (*ajo* is Spanish for *garlic*) with anti-coagulant activity equal or superior to that of aspirin. Raw garlic (three cloves a day) improved clot-dissolving activity by about 20 percent in a double-blind study of medical students in India. Cooking garlic might enhance its anticlotting activity.

Anticancer Effects

Dedicated garlic eaters may escape certain cancers. For example, in a recent study of 42,000 older women in Iowa, those who ate garlic more than once a week were half as likely to develop colon cancer as nongarlic eaters.

Eating just one clove of raw or cooked garlic daily may help protect against stomach and colon cancers. For example, the incidence of stomach cancer is low in a part of Italy where people commonly eat a garlic-rich pesto with their food, compared with other regions where much less garlic is consumed.

Infection Fighter

Garlic kills viruses responsible for colds and the flu, according to tests by James North, a microbiologist at Brigham Young University. Eat garlic when you feel a sore throat coming on, he says, and you may not even get sick. (Eat garlic when you're stuffed up, too; it acts as a decongestant.) Other studies suggest that garlic revs up immune function by stimulating infection-fighting T-cells.

"I recommend eating one or two cloves of raw garlic a day to people with chronic or recurrent infections," says Andrew Weil of the University of Arizona College of Medicine, author of *Natural Health, Natural Medicine*. His tip: Cut raw cloves into small pieces and swallow them like pills.

Effect of Cooking on Garlic's Health Benefits

How you prepare your garlic could affect its health benefits. Researchers from Pennsylvania State University have reported that one minute of microwave heating or 45 minutes of oven roasting can destroy garlic's ability to fight cancer. However, the garlic retained its anticancer abilities if the herb was chopped or crushed and then allowed to stand for 10 minutes before heating. For whole roasted garlic, the anticancer properties can be partially retained if the top of the bulb is sliced off before heating. The 10-minute standing period after chopping or crushing the garlic allows an enzyme, which is destroyed when the garlic is cooked, to produce allyl sulfur compounds with cancer-fighting properties.

Some research suggests that only raw garlic has antibacterial or antiviral effects. (Many of the sauces in this book call for raw garlic. You can also use minced garlic as a garnish.) But both raw and cooked garlic have cardiovascular, decongestive, and anticancer benefits.

For some people, eating raw garlic causes gas, bloating, diarrhea, or even fever. Cooked garlic is gentler on the stomach. All forms of garlic, whether crushed, chopped, stored in jars, prepared in a paste, or even garlic powder off the spice shelf, can have health benefits.

BUYING AND STORING GARLIC

When buying fresh heads of garlic, choose bulbs that are sold loose, not in packages. You need to be able to feel them. Look for large heads that are firm, tight, free of soft spots, and that have an unbroken outer skin. Avoid heads that are dried out or have green sprouts. Garlic sprouts can cause indigestion.

VARIETIES OF GARLIC

Garlic's botanical name is *Allium sativum*. It belongs to the Allium genus, which includes onions, chives, and leeks. A garlic plant will grow from a clove to about 6 inches in height, with spearlike stalks. A head of garlic consists of eight to twenty cloves clustered together in a bulb, and a knot of thin roots at the foot. There are two general varieties of garlic.

Hardneck: This variety has a little stick in the middle (hence the name). It is more difficult to grow, and more perishable. However, hardneck varieties offer a wider range of flavor, and their skin is more colorful. Hardneck garlic is believed to be more closely related to wild garlic.

Softneck: Widely available in supermarkets, softneck varieties contain no hard stick in the center. They are easier to grow and offer the longest shelf life. Their skin is usually white or silvery. Since the stalk is pliable, softneck varieties are used to make garlic braids.

Elephant garlic: Elephant garlic is actually a type of leek, and not true garlic. Elephant garlic has a very mild flavor.

Garlic braids makes a good decoration in your kitchen. However, unless you go through a lot of garlic or have a large family, it is not an economic way to keep garlic around, as the bulbs dry out or sprout before you can use all of them.

Store fresh garlic in a cool, dark place such as a ceramic jar with vent holes, a mesh basket, or a net bag that allows air to circulate around it. Do not store garlic in the refrigerator, where it will absorb moisture.

Unbroken bulbs will normally last for a few months, but once separated from the bulb, the cloves will only last a few weeks or less.

Refrigerating or freezing garlic causes it to lose its fresh flavor. Freezing fresh garlic breaks down its consistency. Peeled garlic cloves stored in the refrigerator can become moldy rather quickly.

Caution: If you make dressings, oils, butters, or marinades containing garlic, be sure to keep them refrigerated at all times, particularly if they are low acid. Otherwise, they pose a threat of potentially deadly botulism. If you leave them out of the refrigerator for even a short while, they should be discarded.

PEELING GARLIC

There are many tools and techniques for peeling garlic. You can use the following methods.

- Place the cloves on a cutting board. Hold a knife flat over the garlic and press down on the blade with your hand, slightly crushing the clove. The skin will crack open and peel off easily.
- Cut the garlic cloves down the middle. It is easy to peel the skin off the halves.
- Use a flexible plastic tube specially designed for peeling garlic. When you roll the garlic in the tube, it rubs off the skin.
- Use a garlic press. Put the clove in the press and squeeze. The garlic flesh comes out and the skin stays in. I have found that unless you are preparing a lot of garlic, the time required for cleaning the press is not worth its use.

Crushed, minced garlic gives out a more pungent, assertive taste than large chunks or whole cloves. The longer you cook the garlic, the milder it tastes.

Because minced garlic only holds its fresh flavor for a few hours, it's best to prepare your garlic ahead of the other ingredients, about ten minutes before you begin to cook.

REMOVING GARLIC ODOR

Garlic has a very strong odor. When you don't want it around, here are a few ways to get rid of it.

From Your Hands

There are hand-deodorizing products you can purchase, but I prefer this simple Asian trick: Soak your hands in a bowl of water that was used to wash rice. The garlic smell vanishes in minutes. You can also rub you hands with fresh ginger or lemon. Follow up by washing with soap and warm water.

From the Cutting Board

Rub the board with a wedge of lemon or a paste of baking soda and water, and rinse. Or simply use the same board to cut more fresh vegetables used in the same recipes, such as cucumbers, tomatoes, and celery.

Soy Foods

My husband, Greg, told me that when he was a child, the soybean was perhaps the most underrated crop in America. While I thrived on soy-based foods along with millions of other Chinese, in the United States soy was grown mainly for its oil and for cattle feed. Or it was plowed under as a green manure crop, to nourish the soil instead of animals or people. Tofu was treated as a joke, something so bland and tasteless that only militant vegetarians ever ate it.

The Chinese approach of saving soybeans for people instead of cattle is a much more efficient use of land and resources. It's much cheaper and easier to grow soy than raise livestock for their protein. These are important considerations in a place like northern China, where land is limited and the climate can be harsh.

Today the United States produces half of the world's soybeans. About 90 percent of that production is still devoted to soy oils and animal feed. The remaining 10 percent goes into an ever-widening array of foods, from breakfast cereals to dairy-free ice cream, and into a wide variety of industrial products. Environmentally friendly newspapers print with soy-based inks. Other products made with soy include paints, soap, and paper.

The first mention of soybeans appears in a description of Chinese plants by the emperor Sheng-Nung from 2838 B.C. From China, soybeans spread to other parts of Asia, and eventually to Europe. By 1765, New England farmers were planting soybeans to make soy sauce and soy noodles for export to England. Yet for the next 150 years, soy crops were primarily grown for oil and the leftover meal was used for animal feed. Early in the twentieth century, scientists began to recognize the nutritional significance of the soybean. Dr. A. A. Horvath, known as the Father of the Soybean, actively promoted soy flour as a protein source for people.

Today, soy is going through a renaissance as Americans discover what Asians have known for thousands of years: Soybeans are more healthful if you eat them than if you feed them to a cow and then eat the cow.

Soy is a complete protein, which means it contains a balanced combination of the essential amino acids you need to stay healthy. It is also an excellent source of iron and B vitamins. Fat content varies, but many soy-based meat substitutes contain less than half the fat of even the leanest ground beef.

Vegetarians find that soy promises more benefits of a vegetarian lifestyle than a diet that relies heavily on grains and starches. Grains and starches contain large amounts of carbohydrates, which can cause hormonal imbalance and make insulin levels soar and blood sugar levels drop quickly. Soy is not only a good protein source for vegetarians, it also decreases their urge to always search for more food to restore blood sugar levels.

As you will discover from the recipes found in this book, soy foods can be delicious and simple to include in your daily diet.

SOY FOODS AND YOUR HEALTH

By the end of the twentieth century, researchers had discovered an astonishing array of health benefits from soy products. Soy now heads a list of "nutraceuticals," foods known to have beneficial pharmacological effects.

This would not surprise the ancient Chinese in the least. The Chinese have long used food as medicine. Chinese medicine considers soy a yin or cooling food. It has been used to treat fevers, headaches, chest distension, hyperactivity, and as a tonic for the lungs and stomach. Here are some of soy's benefits recognized in the West.

Reduces Cancer Risk

Soy foods reduce the risk of breast, colon, and prostate cancer. Rates of prostate cancer mortality are much lower in Asian countries where large amount of soy are consumed. Soybeans contain several naturally occurring compounds, such as phytochemicals like isoflavones, protease inhibitors, and saponins, which seem to protect against the development of cancer. Isoflavones may inhibit enzymes necessary for the growth and spread of many types of cancer.

Lowers Cholesterol Levels

Soybeans are extremely low in saturated fat and free of cholesterol. Research indicates that daily use of soy-based foods may help protect against heart disease by significantly lowering the LDL (bad) cholesterol without reducing the HDL (good) cholesterol levels, even among people with average cholesterol levels.

Prevents Heart Disease

Compounds in soy, such as lecithin, saponins, phytosterols, and isoflavones may favorably affect other risk factors for heart disease beyond cholesterol.

Isoflavones are phytoestrogens, a weak form of estrogen found in soy protein. The two primary isoflavones in soybeans are daidzein and genistein. The potential health benefits of isoflavones are generating interest in the health community. Isoflavones may help to maintain healthy cholesterol levels, which in turn promote overall good health; daidzein has shown promise in this area of study. Given the early stage of research on isoflavones, recommended levels to achieve any beneficial health effects are still under review.

Controls Diabetes

By slowing the absorption of glucose into the bloodstream, soy protects against the damaging effects of high blood glucose levels, common in people with uncontrolled diabetes.

Prevents Osteoporosis

Isoflavones simultaneously increase bone formation while decreasing bone breakdown. Soy protein leads to a lower rate of calcium excretion than protein from animals.

Decreases Menopausal Symptoms

Soy provides a natural source of estrogenlike compounds. Asian women, regular consumers of soy, experience the unpleasant symptoms of menopause like hot flashes and night sweats less often than do western women. Soy may be the reason.

BUYING AND STORING SOY

Increasing varieties of soy foods can be found in health food stores, or the natural foods section of many grocery stores. Asian markets are a great resource for traditional soy foods. Soy foods range from traditional tofu, tempeh, and miso to innovative soy-based cheese, yogurt, and ice cream. Soy-based meat substitutes can replace burgers, hot dogs, sausage, bacon, fish, and chicken. Last year my family celebrated Thanksgiving with a tofu turkey that we bought at the local health food store.

Soy products are sold fresh, frozen, canned, or dried. With so many alternatives on the market, be aware that they are not all health promoting. A few of them are high in sodium and contain monosodium glutamate (MSG). Read the label before purchasing. Buy organic products to avoid pesticides and herbicides.

Always refrigerate or freeze fresh soy products. After opening canned foods, place leftovers in sealed containers and refrigerate. Don't store foods in metal cans. Store dry products in a cool and dry place.

COOKING WITH SOY

The Buddhist vegetarian diet has led to the creation of an amazing variety of soy products. Many times I have attended vegetarian banquets in Asia. The substitutes for chicken, duck, fish, shrimp, and squid taste like the real thing, or even better. Soy products are very versatile. Due to its mild taste, it can be easily paired with other ingredients.

Soy foods can be used in soups, stir-fried or grilled, baked, or even steamed. See the individual soy products for suggestions. Use firm tofu or dense soy products for grilling and stir-frying and for dishes that require a longer cooking time. Add soft tofu to fast-cooking dishes and drinks.

Soy is considered a yin food. When you cook soy, think about flavoring it with yang ingredients such as ginger, garlic, and chili peppers for balance.

Shiitake Mushrooms

While there are many varieties of mushrooms, I focus on shiitake mushrooms because they have been subjected to the most research on their health benefits, and they are one of the most popular kinds. The shiitake mushroom is called the king of mushrooms.

Shiitake mushrooms are native to Asia. In the wild, the "*take*" or mushroom grows on the trunks of fallen Japanese *shii* trees. So *shiitake* translates to "*shii* tree mushroom." It also grows well on other broad-leaved trees, including many native North American species. This allowed American farmers to quickly enter the shiitake market when this mushroom started to become popular in the United States.

Wild shiitake takes up to six years for the shiitake fungus *Lentinus edodes* to produce mushroom fruit. While some growers continue growing shiitake on logs, others reduce the growing time to just a few months. They do this by first creating their own logs or blocks. The blocks can be made of sawdust or wood shavings. Some growers add other ingredients such as grains to the block. They sterilize the blocks and then inoculate them with actively growing fungus, or spawn. The shiitake spawn takes off and produces mushrooms in as little as three months.

SHIITAKE MUSHROOMS AND YOUR HEALTH

The Chinese as well as the Japanese and Koreans have prized shiitake's taste and reputed medicinal benefits for over two thousand years. In traditional Chinese medicine, shiitake is important for stimulating the *qi* or life force and it is considered a neutral food. It was believed to be essential for a long and healthy life and was prescribed for a wide range of ailments such as fatigue, arthritis, colds, gastrointestinal problems, liver ailments, and vision problems.

Lentinan is a component of shiitake that is believed to strengthen the immune system and destroy cancerous and virus-infected cells. It helps prolong the survival time of cancer patients by supporting the immune system. Lentinan may also prevent the increase of chromosomal damage induced by anticancer drugs. Lentinan is administered in Japan to cancer patients as an adjunct to chemotherapy. HIV patients may also benefit from lentinan, which is commercially available for clinical use. It is one of the top-selling anticancer drugs in Japan.

A compound called eritadenine and the dietary fiber present in shiitake help increase the rate at which cholesterol is excreted from the body. Other compounds may lower blood pressure, thin the blood, and prevent abnormal clotting—all beneficial to the heart and circulation.

Shiitake mushrooms contain all eight essential amino acids along with glutamic acid, which is important for the brain.

Shiitake mushrooms are low in calories and a good source of dietary fiber. They are a rich source of minerals and vitamins A, B_2, B_{12}, C; niacin; and ergosterol (a vitamin D precursor). All these attributes make shiitake an excellent addition to a healthy diet.

BUYING AND STORING SHIITAKE MUSHROOMS

You can find two forms of shiitake mushrooms in the store: fresh and dried.

Fresh Mushrooms

When shopping for fresh shiitake, look for firm caps that are fleshy, plump, and dry. Avoid withered or slimy caps.

One fun alternative for getting fresh mushrooms is to grow your own. Many growers provide kits by mail order or over the Internet. With proper care you can harvest your own fresh mushrooms in just a few weeks.

Fresh mushrooms should be refrigerated in a paper bag, or wrapped in a dry paper towel and placed in a plastic bag in the refrigerator. They will last up to five days.

Dried Mushrooms

Dried shiitake comes in different grades of quality. Look for intact mushrooms that have thick caps.

Dried shiitake will keep indefinitely if stored in a cool, dark place or in the freezer.

PREPARING AND COOKING SHIITAKE MUSHROOMS

I use fresh mushrooms more often because I prefer the taste of fresh mushrooms over dried, and because fresh mushrooms are becoming more readily available.

To prepare fresh shiitake mushrooms: Rinse in cold water to wash off any sand or dirt. Pay extra attention to the gills. Trim off the woody stems and set them aside for use in mushroom stock or broth.

Dried shiitake mushrooms can be used in recipes calling for fresh ones but first they need to be soaked. The hydrated mushrooms can be sliced, minced, chopped, or used in their entirety. First, soak the mushrooms in hot water until they soften, about 15 minutes. (Soaking time varies with type and size.) Rinse the gills (the underside) under running water to clean them of any dirt or sand. Squeeze the mushrooms in your hand to thoroughly wring out the water. Remove and discard tough, woody stems.

Fresh shiitake mushrooms are very versatile. You can sauté, broil, or bake them. The stems add a wonderful flavor to soup stock.

- Sautéing or stir-frying: Slice the mushrooms into thin strips and sauté or stir-fry in a little oil or broth until tender, 1 to 2 minutes.
- Grilling or broiling: Marinate large whole mushroom caps in an herbed vinaigrette or broth. Place on the grill or under the broiler and cook for 2 to 3 minutes, or until soft and tender. Turn the mushrooms as they color.
- Braising: Heat a little vegetable or chicken broth, add chopped garlic,

ginger, and/or chilies and whole mushroom caps, and either cook slowly on top of the stove or oven-braise at 375°F (190°C) for 10 minutes, until tender. Turn the mushrooms halfway through cooking. Serve with remaining pan juices.

- Simmering: Use whole or sliced mushroom caps in soups and stews. In soups, drop mushrooms into simmering soup and cook until tender. In stews, add mushrooms when adding other vegetables and simmer until stew is done.
- Fillings: Mince mushrooms caps and mix with other filling for meatball or dumpling fillings.

Ginseng

Fresh in my memory, I can still see a tall, red wooden dresser, on top of which sat a cardboard box decorated with delicate patterns. Inside the box was a whole wild ginseng root wrapped with red silk. This was in my grandmother's room. I was only allowed to see the ginseng when Grandmother showed it to her guests. The ginseng was shaped like a man. A couple of times I was even allowed to touch the "head." My grandmother told me that ginseng would keep a person away from all sickness and bring peace and happiness to the soul.

I first ate ginseng at a young age, not in the form of a pill or tea, but cooked with food. I was taught to respect and value ginseng. Each root has its own character and personality. In China, ginseng was and is expensive. It is considered an exotic and valuable plant. When available, it is first given to the old and sick. Thanks to a relative who worked on a ginseng farm in the famous Changbai Shan Mountains in northeast China, Grandmother received ginseng for her old age. I got to eat some because I was her favorite granddaughter.

In Chinese, ginseng is called *renshen*, which means, "root of person." It is the most widely recognized medicinal plant in Chinese medicine. There are many varieties of ginseng, but they all belong to the small botanical family called Araliaceae.

Ginseng roots often grow into shapes that resemble a humanlike figure, which is why they got their name. The mature root is more valuable than a younger one. The more mature the root, the more humanlike its shape and the higher its value. Ginseng grows wild and is also cultivated. Some varieties of wild ginseng are very rare and hard to find. For that reason, the price gap between wild and cultivated products is very large. The majority of ginseng products we find on the market today are cultivated.

GINSENG AND YOUR HEALTH

There are numerous types of ginseng supplements on the market. I have been asked many times, "Why do the Chinese take ginseng? How do they take it? What is the difference between the many types of ginseng? Can ginseng supplements give me energy so I can work longer and sleep less?" I will try to answer these questions in this book and share with you some of my favorite traditional family ginseng recipes.

Ginseng plays a major role in the concept of yin and yang. If one's balance is disturbed, a suitable type of ginseng is used to restore the body's balance. When one feels a lack of energy, he would be in an excess yin condition, and he would need to take "hot" ginseng as a stimulant. If one is feeling hyperactive, she is in an excess yang condition and needs to take "cool" ginseng to strengthen her yin. To maintain a balanced system and increase stamina, one may want to turn to neutral ginseng.

The active ingredients in ginseng are called saponins. The saponins in Asian and American ginseng are called ginsenosides. The saponins in Siberian ginseng are called eleutherosides. These chemicals help our body adapt and adjust to many potentially harmful agents.

Like many herbs, ginseng can be a powerful healing agent when used properly. It is important to understand the concept of yin and yang and choose the type of ginseng that fits your needs. Since ginseng's species vary slightly in composition and effect, the following information may help you to determine what type of ginseng to use. The two main factors are season of the year and the individual's needs.

If you want to use ginseng as medicine, talk to a reputable Chinese herbalist about combining ginseng with different Chinese herbal formulas to treat various diseases. As always, be sure to inform your medical doctor before adding new treatments to your regimen.

While there are many different types of ginseng, the three most commonly used ginseng varieties are Asian, American, and Siberian.

Asian Ginseng

Asian ginseng (*Panax ginseng C. A. Meyer*) was named after botanist C. A. Meyer, who first identified it in the early eighteenth century. This species is native primarily to China and Korea. Dried peeled ginseng root is called "white ginseng." A steamed, unpeeled ginseng root is called "red ginseng," because the steaming process turns the root red. Don't eat Asian ginseng when you have a flu or fever.

Asian ginseng has a yang effect. It is warm and stimulating. It has too much heat to be used in warm months. It is better to use it in winter.

Asian ginseng boosts energy and vitality. It is used by sick, older persons; women after giving birth; postmenopausal women; and vegetarians. Since vegetarians lack the yang found in red meat, in general they need more yang in their systems. Some Chinese doctors believe Asian ginseng is best for a person over forty-five years old. It is also used for lack of sleep, overwork, low energy, low motivation, and mild depression.

Chinese ginseng whole roots and slices have a sweet, mild taste.

American Ginseng

Jesuit missionaries discovered American ginseng (*Panax quinquefolius*) in the 1700s and 1800s. It was growing wild in the northern United States, particularly in Wisconsin, and in Canada. It is the closest cousin to Asian ginseng and looks like a compact version of it. Native Americans used it long before the continent was colonized. By the late eighteenth century, wild ginseng was becoming rare and cultivation began. Today, American ginseng products are made from one- to five-year-old cultivated ginseng.

American ginseng has a yin effect; it is cool and relaxing. It regulates metabolism, increasing fluids. It is suited for younger, hotter, more energetic people—athletes; women during menopause; hyperactive or stressed persons; and nonvegetarians. It is used to treat fevers and what Chinese herbal doctors call "yin-deficient ailments." Due to its cooling effect, American ginseng is good in the summer.

American whole roots and slices have a mild flavor. Fresh ones have an earthy taste.

Siberian Ginseng

Siberian ginseng (*Eleutherococcus senticosus*) grows mainly in the northern tundra regions of eastern Russia. It is not a member of the *Panax* genus but still belongs to the family. Technically it is not ginseng but has similar effects to true ginseng. When true ginseng became expensive and hard to find, Russians used it as an alternative. Its root requires days of soaking and cooking, due to the tough fiber. In this book we are going to use only the tea, not the root, for cooking.

Siberian ginseng is neither yin or yang; it is neutral. It maintains a balanced system, increases energy and stamina, and supports weak lungs and heart. It is widely used by athletes and performers in Russia. Siberian ginseng can be used year-round. It has a smoky, sweet taste.

BUYING AND STORING GINSENG

Ginseng comes in the form of fresh or dried whole roots, minced or powdered dry roots, and fresh or dry slices.

Whole Roots

Look for a root that is at least four years old to get the full ginseng benefits. If you are willing to pay the price, wild ones are better than cultivated ones, but the cultivated ones will give you enough health benefits. There are two harvest seasons for ginseng: One is after the snows melt in the spring, between March and May; the other is in the fall between September and November. Those are the best times to buy fresh ginseng roots. Be sure to wash the fresh ginseng before using—a lot of roots will still have some grit.

Fresh roots and slices: Dry the ginseng with paper towels. Place it in a sealed brown paper bag in the refrigerator. Or wrap the roots in paper towels and seal in a plastic bag stored in the refrigerator. Be sure to check the towels periodically. If they get moist, change the towels to prevent rotting. Place the ginseng in a separate section of the refrigerator so it will not absorb flavors from other foods. It can last up to two months. You can also divide the ginseng into serving sizes, place the servings in individual sealed plastic bags, and store in the freezer for up to a year. Don't refreeze the ginseng once it's thawed.

Dried ginseng roots or slices: The Chinese prefer to bury whole roots in their rice jar, a very large glazed ceramic jar. If you have one in your home, I recommend you take advantage of it. Just make sure you remember to find it later. The rice absorbs moisture and prevents the ginseng from becoming moist, which will cause bacterial growth and rot the ginseng. It will last five years or longer. You can also store it the modern way—in a sealed glass jar in a cool, dry place. It can last up to five years. After that, the roots may get too dry and start to lose their health benefits. Don't refrigerate dry ginseng for long periods of time. This could cause the ginseng to lose too much moisture.

Minced and Powdered Dry Roots

Mature ginseng looks like a person. Often tea and powder are made from what would be the feet, arms, and head of the "person" and any additional side roots off the main body. The most common forms are ginseng tea, ginseng powder, and sliced ginseng.

Ginseng tea: Made with minced ginseng root, it is one of the most widely available forms on the market. Be sure to find a product that is made with pure root, not with ginseng leaves and other ingredients. It is suitable for salad dressings, sauces, soups, stir-frying, and of course, drinking.

Ginseng powder: Made with mashed/ground ginseng root, ginseng powder comes in the form of bottled ginseng powder or as a pill. Find a product that is made with pure root, not mixed with other ingredients. If you have a difficult time locating powdered ginseng, you can open a ginseng capsule, use the powder inside, and discard the shell. It is suitable for steamed buns, breads, sauces, and soups. Ginseng powder of any variety tends to taste bitter and strong.

Sliced ginseng: You can get slices in a dry form. The more mature and larger the diameter of the root slice, the better. You can also buy the ginseng root and slice it yourself. Sliced ginseng is good for use in soups, hot pots, sauces, and stir-fried foods.

Minced and Powdered Ginseng

Unopened packages can be stored in a cool, dry place. Open packages should be stored in a tightly sealed glass jar or a sealed plastic bag in the refrigerator. Depending on the product and packaging, in general, both methods can keep ginseng products two years or longer. Be sure to check the manufacturer's expiration date.

Ginseng Stored in Alcohol

If you go to the home of an older Chinese person, chances are you are going to see whole ginseng roots soaking in a bottle of alcohol. Chinese believe it is good for blood circulation and to rejuvenate the body.

Place about 1 to 2 ounces of whole fresh ginseng in a bottle of alcohol, such as Chinese red sorghum wine, liqueur, whiskey, or sake. Seal tightly. Let it soak for 10 days or longer. Drink with meals or use for cooking.

COOKING WITH GINSENG

In China, cooking a whole ginseng root, especially a wild one, is viewed as an important event. Many times, the family performs complicated ceremonies. First, they light incense sticks to pay respect to their ancestors and to thank them for the good fortune in receiving the ginseng. The diners fast for three or four days to cleanse their bodies before consuming the root. During the fast they drink chrysanthemum tea to help open the meridians (lines of energy within the body). Food preparations may run from simple chicken soup and tea made with the ginseng, to a whole feast. To get all the benefits from the root, it is cooked a long time and eaten at the end of the meal.

For cooking, I have found that ginseng tea and slices are the most convenient. Some recipes call for the whole root, but the root requires more time to prepare. It is also more expensive than other forms. If you ever come across a recipe that calls for whole ginseng root, feel free to substitute sliced ginseng. If you are using a dry form when the recipe calls for minced ginseng slices, soak the slices in hot water to soften before cutting. Be sure to drink the liquid while you cook.

Ginseng is not an instant miracle cure. It is a good idea to start out slowly and to take it on a regular basis, rather than a large amount over a short period. The Chinese use ginseng to gradually restore yin/yang balance, and too much of the wrong kind can further upset the balance. It is possible to have too much of a good thing. As with any supplement, you should start with a small amount. If you feel you are getting some benefits, then you can gradually increase your quantity. The amount of ginseng cooked with food in this book is small, which will not give you obvious benefits or cure any disease in a short time. After all, as an old Chinese saying goes, "Train your soldiers a thousand days for one war." The aim is to build up a long-term health effect and to give your food a wonderfully exotic, additional flavor. You can choose the type of ginseng—Asian, American, or Siberian—based on your own needs.

According to Chinese doctors, you should avoid cooking Asian ginseng with carrots, turnips, and radishes. These mustard-family vegetables are exhausting and conflict with the positive yang aspects of ginseng.

I recommend the following amounts for cooking. The amounts are small, but add flavor to your food. Eat it regularly and increase usage gradually. Give your body a chance to get used to ginseng's health effects. Only use the ginseng powder when other forms are not available, as it has a much stronger taste.

- Add 1 ounce fresh or dry root for stock and soup.
- Use 6 ginseng slices, about 0.25 ounce, or 2 ginseng tea bags to brew each cup of tea for cooking (each ginseng tea bag contains about 1 teaspoon of ginseng).
- Brew ¼ teaspoon ginseng powder (amount in each pill) in 1 cup of water.

Green Tea

Just as Americans grow up drinking a variety of fruit juices, I grew up drinking a variety of teas. I also ate many dishes prepared with tea. Yes, "ate." The Chinese have been cooking with green tea almost as long as they have been drinking it.

The Chinese have consumed tea since A.D. 800. For centuries we have revered it as a natural healer for body and soul.

All true traditional teas come from the *Camellia sinensis* plant. Newly plucked leaves, considered "natural" or "fresh," are the source of the dried tea. The quality of a tea depends on the quality and condition of the fresh leaves: the younger the leaves of the plant, the higher their quality. The processing of tea, by inducing physical or chemical changes in the leaf, produces the three major types. Black tea is made from fully fermented leaves. Oolong or red tea is partially fermented, and its flavor and color fall between black tea and green tea. Green tea is made from unfermented leaves.

In addition to the main types of tea, there are flavored teas, made by the addition of other plant leaves, flowers, roots, fruit, or spices to the tea leaves.

Herbal teas are made of other plant leaves, flowers, roots, or spices, but do not contain real tea.

GREEN TEA AND YOUR HEALTH

Recently, researchers have found that green tea is a natural source of antioxidants. The antioxidants may have important health benefits. They prevent or delay damage to your body's cells and tissues. They reduce the risk of having a heart attack and protect the blood vessels that feed your heart and brain.

Hot and chilled green teas contain the same amount of antioxidant, but not the bottled ones. A study funded by the United States Department of Agriculture (USDA) found that bottled teas lack the major antioxidants, and some are loaded with sugar.

Researchers at the University of Kansas attributed to green tea one hundred times the antioxidant strength of vitamin C, and twenty-five times that of vitamin E. Another USDA study found that the antioxidant capacity of green tea is better than that of twenty-two various fruits and vegetables. A study conducted by the USDA Human Nutrition Research Center on Aging found that 1 cup of tea brewed for 3 to 5 minutes contains about the same amount of antioxidants as one serving of vegetables.

One cup of regular green tea contains only about one-third the caffeine in a cup of coffee. Decaffeinated tea contains nearly as many antioxidants as regular tea.

Researchers at Case Western Reserve University found that green tea may prevent inflammation from injury or from diseases such as arthritis. The antioxidants in green tea inhibit the Cox-2 enzyme, which causes inflammation.

Green tea may prevent skin cancer. Research at the University Hospital of Cleveland found that skin damage from ultraviolet light was lower when the skin was protected by green tea.

Purdue University researchers found that green tea leaves are rich in EGCG, a compound that inhibits an enzyme required for cancer cell growth, and that can kill cultured cancer cells with no ill effect on healthy cells. According to Purdue University researchers Dorothy Morre and D. James Morre, green tea leaves are rich in a compound that inhibits the growth of cancer cells.

Green tea has also been found to regulate blood cholesterol and blood sugar levels, lower blood pressure, fight aging, increase immunity, and promote weight loss.

According to Dr. Lester A. Mitscher, chair of the medical chemistry department at Kansas University and the author of *The Green Tea Book*, "The polyphenols—antioxidants found in green tea—have been found to be among the most effective antioxidants, more powerful than vitamins C and E." Dr. Mitscher recommends that people consume the equivalent of at least 4 cups of green tea per day to maximize its health benefits.

With the fast pace of life today, I find it hard to make the time for 4 cups of green tea every day. The Chinese solution is to incorporate green tea into cooking. You too can enjoy not only the unique flavor it brings to cooking, but a healthier mind and body.

BREWING TEA

According to the American Tea Council, tea is regularly consumed by more than half the population in the United States. Eighty percent of tea is steeped from tea bags, while the rest of it is brewed from loose tea. Some dedicated tea drinkers insist that loose leaf renders the finest flavor and aroma. Most of us may be hard-pressed to tell the difference.

Never boil water for tea in an aluminum teakettle, or steep tea in plastic or aluminum. Stainless steel is nonreactive and does not absorb flavor or odors, thus providing the purest water for tea.

I prefer to brew tea in Yixing teapots, which have been used in China since the Sung Dynasty (960–1279). These pots are made of purple clay enriched with natural minerals. The pot develops a rich patina and "seasoning" with use that enhances the taste and aroma to bring out the best of a fine tea.

Other good choices for teapots are china, porcelain, and stainless steel. Always fill your teacup or teapot with hot water to preheat it and discard the water before adding the tea and the brewing water. Covering the teapot or cup helps the tea leaves unfurl, which also helps loose tea leaves settle to the bottom.

Fresh bottled spring water is the best choice for making tea. The second choice would be filtered water. Tap water contains chemicals that can alter the taste of a brew. Different types of tea require different temperatures of water.

For the best flavor and the most infusions, brew green tea with water at 160° to 170°F (71° to 76°C). This is when the water first begins to stir. It's restless but not simmering. It is better to steep green tea at a lower temperature for a little longer than to force the leaves to give up their essence with high temperatures, which will end up making a bitter brew. According to research, after 3 to 4 minutes of brewing time, you will get all the health benefits from the green tea.

COOKING WITH GREEN TEA

After I came to America, I found myself using tea bags instead of loose tea. According to research, the finer the green tea, the more health benefits you get. Since the tea in a bag is finely chopped, you may get more benefits by using tea bags.

In this book, I brewed from tea bags for soup bases, marinades, and sauces. To get the most of green tea's delicate flavor and health benefits, I use two to three times as much tea as for making tea for drinking.

To use the tea from teabags for seasoning: Cut open the fresh teabags and remove the contents, discarding the empty bags. Heat a wok or frying pan with oil. Add the tea and cook until the tea releases its flavor before adding the rest of the ingredients.

When a recipe calls for loose tea, you can also substitute tea leaves from tea bags in most instances. Because the tea in teabags is finer than loose tea, there are some recipes where only loose tea will work. In recipes in which loose tea is required, I have indicated such. Two tea bags are equal to about ½ tablespoon loose tea.

Brewing Tea Bags for Cooking

Warm the teapot or cup by swirling a little steaming water in it. Discard the water. Place 2 to 4 tea bags into the pot. Immediately pour 1 cup boiling water over the tea bags. Cover, infuse for 5 to 7 minutes. Discard the tea bags. This makes 1 cup of very strong tea. Use this liquid according to the recipes.

Brewing Tea Leaves for Cooking

The Chinese have been cooking with high-quality green tea leaves for centuries. We use dry leaves as a seasoning, the brew as a sauce base, and the infused leaves as vegetables. I have found that the best tea for using as a vegetable is Dragon Well; the best type to use as a seasoning is gunpowder, and any fine green tea is good for brewing tea for the soup base.

When using as a seasoning, add the dry leaves to the heated oil like any other seasoning. Use green tea sauces for marinades, cooking, and dipping. When cooking with tea leaves, we first brew or steam the leaves. When brewing we need the leaves fully infused, so don't use a tea ball or infusing basket. Try to think of the tea leaves as a delicate leafy vegetable. Another way to infuse tea leaves is to steam them until infused before adding to the dish.

Infusing Tea Leaves to Use as a Vegetable

Warm the teapot or cup by swirling steaming water in it. Discard the water. Place 1 teaspoon loose tea into the pot. Immediately pour ½ cup boiling water over the tea. Cover and let the leaves infuse for 4 to 5 minutes. This will make 1 tablespoon infused leaves. Save the liquid for a sauce and use the leaves for cooking.

2. Cooking Basics

I enjoy experimenting in the kitchen and creating new dishes. Good equipment not only makes cooking easy and fun, but also adds enjoyment to my daily life. Did I mention before that I love good food? If you are tired of eating the same dishes week after week, here is a new beginning. The following equipment is not a must but can definitely reduce your time in the kitchen, make life more exciting, and win you praise at the dinner table.

Equipment

INDOOR AND OUTDOOR GRILLS

Stovetop Grilling Pan

This is a frying pan with parallel ridges on the bottom. It comes in round and square shapes. Since less of the food's surface comes in contact with the pan and its nonstick surface, you need less oil. The ridges create searing and simulate grill marks while the flavorful juices remain in the pan, keeping the food moist and tender. Grilled food requires less seasoning. Even better, I can grill all year round, even when a big snowstorm hits Colorado. A lid and a kitchen fan help reduce smoke to a minimum. (The lid for my 12-inch wok fits my grilling pan.)

REFRIGERATORS

WHENEVER I DO A COOKING CLASS, I AM USUALLY ASKED WHAT KIND OF REFRIGERATOR ONE SHOULD HAVE. BECAUSE A REFRIGERATOR IS ON ALL THE TIME, IT CONSUMES MORE ELECTRICITY THAN ANY OTHER HOUSEHOLD APPLIANCE. (IT IS NOT NECESSARILY RUNNING ALL THE TIME, IT RUNS ONLY WHEN THE THERMOSTAT CALLS FOR THE COMPRESSOR TO TURN ON, WHICH CAN VARY DRAMATICALLY ACCORDING TO USAGE OF THE UNIT.) IN ADDITION TO CONSIDERING THE SIZE, COLOR, STYLE AND OTHER FEATURES, ONE IMPORTANT THING TO LOOK FOR IS THE ENERGY STAR LABEL, WHICH CAN SAVE YOU A LOT OF MONEY OVER THE LIFE OF THE APPLIANCE. (THE ENERGY STAR LABEL IS THE GOVERNMENT'S SEAL OF APPROVAL. IT WAS CREATED BY THE U.S. DEPARTMENT OF ENERGY AND THE U.S. ENVIRONMENTAL PROTECTION AGENCY TO IDENTIFY THE MOST ENERGY-EFFICIENT PRODUCTS ON THE MARKET. ENERGY STAR–LABELED APPLIANCES EXCEED EXISTING FEDERAL EFFICIENCY STANDARDS BY AT LEAST 10 PERCENT.)

THERE ARE TWO TYPES OF REFRIGERATORS, FREE-STANDING AND BUILT-IN. FREE-STANDING UNITS ARE WHAT MOST AMERICANS ARE FAMILIAR WITH AND CAN BE EASILY MOVED AND FIT INTO EXISTING AREAS WITHOUT ANY CABINETRY WORK. BUILT-IN REFRIGERATORS, AS THE NAME IMPLIES, REQUIRE CUSTOMIZED CABINETRY TO MAKE THE REFRIGERATOR LOOK "BUILT-IN" TO THE SURROUNDING CABINETS. THESE UNITS CAN VARY DRAMATICALLY IN SIZE FROM 36" WIDE TO 72".

THERE ARE THREE STYLES OF REFRIGERATORS: TWO-DOOR WITH A TOP FREEZER, SIDE-BY-SIDE WITH DOORS OPENING IN THE CENTER, AND TWO-DOOR WITH A BOTTOM FREEZER. GENERALLY, THE MODELS WITH THE FREEZER ON THE TOP ARE MOST ENERGY EFFICIENT.

Outdoor Gas Grill

There are many gas grills on the market with prices ranging from $150 to thousands of dollars. If you think like the Chinese, you want to get the best deal for the least money. Find a high-quality grill that will last for years rather than a cheap one, which you will need to replace after a couple of seasons. It will save you money and time in the end.

Look at and compare the following features when choosing a gas grill:

- Size of the cooking surface
- Number of burners
- Extra features: side burner, rotisserie, side shelves, wheels
- Materials: stainless steel components—rustproof and easier to clean than cast iron
- Number of years in the warranty
- Appearance and color
- Cover—to protect your grill if it remains outdoors year-round

ICE-CREAM MAKERS

Bucket Ice-Cream Makers

In general, you can make more ice cream with the bucket models, but they require ice and salt. Ice and salt help lower the temperature. Their operation can get messy. Unless you are making ice cream for a big party, you end up with one flavor of ice cream for a long time. They are available in manual and electric models. The advantage of the manual ones is that you can get the kids involved—my son loves to help make ice cream almost as much as he enjoys eating it.

Cylinder Ice-Cream Makers

Cylinder makers require no salt and ice. All you need to do is remember to place the cylinder in your freezer the night before. The cylinder contains a liquid coolant, which will chill your ice cream. During the summer I tend to leave the cylinder in my freezer most of the time. When I am short of freezer space I simply tuck my frozen vegetables or other food into the cylinder's bowl. Cylinders are available in manual and electric models.

WOKS

I can't imagine a kitchen without a wok. It is so versatile. You can use it to stir-fry, steam, and even cook soup. I "store" mine near my stove. It is worth paying a little bit more to get a high-quality wok. The nonstick coating on cheaper ones tends to peel after a period of use, and the coating may get into your food. If you don't have a wok, don't let that stop you from cooking. A chef's pan or a large, deep skillet can work just as well. Be sure to buy one that is nonstick.

STEAMERS

When you want a flavorful, healthy meal, what could be better than steaming? It brings out all the original flavor of the food with little effort. Steam food by suspending it over boiling water. It is an excellent method of cooking low-fat yet delicious food. You can choose from many types of steamers on the market. Or, as I tell my husband whenever he wants to buy a new power tool, "Make use of existing resources." Chances are you already have one of the following steamer solutions in your kitchen. If not, look for a steamer big enough to meet your needs. For a single person, a vegetable steam rack will do. For a larger family, you may need a stacking steamer rack that will fit on your largest cooking pot.

Be sure to always lift the cover up away from you so your hand is not exposed to the scalding steam. Check the water level often. Replenish the water as necessary. Be sure the food remains above the water level and is not submerged.

Using a Wok as a Steamer

You will need a metal vegetable steaming rack and a lid. To prevent the metal rack from scratching the bottom of a nonstick wok, set the rack on a heatproof plate. If you don't have any kind of rack, use a small bowl filled with water, and place a plate of food on top. Fill your wok about one-third full with hot water and bring to a boil. Cover and steam.

Using a Large Pot as a Steamer

I like a steam rack that fits snugly over the top of the pot. If you are steaming a small amount of food, you don't need a deep pot or a lot of water. Just make sure there's enough water to keep the food steaming until done. You may want a teakettle of hot water close at hand in case you need to add more. If you are stacking three steam racks on top of the pot, you need a deep pot with a lot of water, perhaps two-thirds full, to provide the power needed to steam all that food. Once the water reaches a rolling boil, stack all the steam racks over the pot and cover with a lid. This way you can steam a couple of dishes at a time.

If you have a folding steam basket, place a heatproof bowl in the bottom of the pot within about 2 inches of the hot water. Place the food in a heatproof bowl or plate that will fit in the basket. Bring the water to a boil. Put the plate of food on the steam basket.

Using a European Steamer

If you have a metal steamer that is wide enough to take a plate of food, this will produce the same results as any other steamer. Be sure the food stays a few inches above the boiling water.

Steaming Leftovers: Steaming is one of the best methods of reheating food. It warms food without cooking it further, and puts back some moisture. To reheat rice, noodles and braised dishes, bring the water to a simmer but do not boil. Steam the food over medium-low heat to prevent overcooking.

SKILLETS

Skillets are shallow pans with one long handle, but you may also hear them called frying pans, sauté pans, omelet pans, or gourmet pans. The ones with low, sloped sides are best for pan-frying and omelets; higher, straight sides are best for stir-frying or cooking dishes with lots of liquid. Skillets come in sizes ranging from 7 to 14 inches in diameter. If you want only one, buy an all-purpose size—10 or 12 inches, preferably a nonstick one with a cover.

RICE COOKER

I use my rice cooker more often than any other kitchen appliance. There are a variety of sizes and styles on the market. Find a size that fits your family's needs, with a non-stick cooking pan that prevents rice from sticking and ensures fast and easy cleanup. A good feature to look for is an automatic warming system that will keep your rice warm and moist for up to twelve hours.

KNIVES

No tool is more important in the kitchen than a good, quality knife. It will save you time and make cooking more enjoyable. The key is to find a set of knives that fits your hand and feels comfortable to use day after day. I find large and heavy knives are too much to handle. My eight-inch chef's knife is the one I use the most. It is worth buying high-quality knives rather than low-quality ones that dull quickly.

Techniques

Many of the following techniques are used throughout this book. Mastering the basic skills will make it easier to cook healthy and quick meals.

CUTTING TECHNIQUES

When you slice and shred, the objective is to create uniform-size pieces that will cook evenly. Seasoning ingredients and garnishes such as herbs should be minced. Mincing makes the ingredients small enough to cook all the flavor into the dish, or to give the dish a light touch of color.

Slicing: Hold the food firmly on the cutting board with one hand while the other hand holds the knife firmly. Cut the food straight down into very thin slices.

Shredding: Cut the food into ⅛-inch slices, then stack several slices and cut them lengthwise into ⅛-inch-thick matchstick-size pieces.

Mincing: Shred the food, then dice the shreds. One hand firmly holds the knife handle while the other holds down the blunt edge of the knife blade. Rock the knife up and down to mince the food evenly.

GARNISHING

This is the final touch to ensure your creation becomes a masterpiece. Keep it simple. Even two sprigs of cilantro or a sprinkling of minced red bell pepper adds an artistic finish to the dish.

MIXING SAUCES

Many recipes in this book call for a sauce to be added to the dish. Always prepare the sauce before you start cooking. Make sure the mixture is smooth and well blended before adding it to the dish. For dipping sauces, the longer the dry ingredients marinate, the stronger the flavor will be. Refrigerate sauces in a sealed container.

SIMMERING

This technique is used for soups, sauces, and stews. Simmering is a slow-cooking process that helps the food absorb more flavor from the other ingredients, as well as the sauce. Immerse the food in just enough boiling water to cover it. Bring the water back to a boil and then reduce the temperature below the boiling point.

STEAMING

Steaming is the second most widely used cooking method in China. Steamed food is cooked by suspending the food over boiling water. It is an excellent method of cooking low-fat—yet delicious—food.

When steaming food, check the water level often and replenish the water as necessary. The food must remain above the water level and not get wet. When lifting the lid during steaming, always lift it up away from you so your hand is not exposed to the scalding steam.

STIR-FRYING

Stir-frying is the most common Chinese cooking technique. It is also a good way to cook healthy and fast meals. With a nonstick wok or cooking pan, you need very little oil. Most stir-fried dishes take only minutes to prepare. Because the cooking time is short, the food retains its natural flavors, nutrients, and textures.

Stir-frying can be a little intimidating at first. The following steps will ensure your successful and safe stir-frying.

Prepare the ingredients correctly: To ensure even and fast cooking, most of these recipes call for thinly sliced or shredded ingredients. This is when you will appreciate a good set of knives. I use chopping as a form of meditation. Put on some classical music, and chop, chop, chop. If you don't have time or have your own form of meditation, don't let that stop you from stir-frying. You can always use pre-cut meats, bagged salad, and even frozen vegetables. That is what I do many weeknights.

Assemble all the ingredients: Stir-frying is like a roller-coaster ride—once you start, there's no stopping. So make sure you have everything cut, meats marinated, and sauces mixed. Arrange everything near the wok, including the serving plate and garnishes.

Set the table: That's right! Stir-fried food tastes its best when it is hot. You don't want your hot creation getting cold and soggy. (If dinner is delayed, place the food in a covered dish and keep it warm in an oven set on warm.)

Order of cooking: Stir-frying is usually done in batches, and the order in which ingredients are added is important. Aromatic seasonings like green tea, ginger, and garlic usually go in first, followed by meats or seafood, and hard vegetables such as carrots go in before softer ones such as spinach. Add the sauce when all the food is halfway cooked.

Begin to cook: Use high heat. Heat the wok or cooking pan for 30 seconds before adding the oil. Drizzle in the oil, usually no more than 2 tablespoons. Swirl it to coat the surface. Don't wait until the oil is too hot. If you hold your hand above the wok and can feel the heat, it's ready. If the recipe calls for dry green tea leaves, garlic, ginger, or chili pepper, this is the time to add it. With practice you can judge cooking time by the food's sound and smell. The purpose here is to flavor the oil and release the fragrance of the seasonings. Quickly add other ingredients and cover immediately to prevent splattering. Keep the food moving by giving the wok a couple of good shakes. After a couple seconds of shaking, you are safe to open the lid and start stir-frying. Most of the water will have cooked off.

Stir: Use your spatula to toss the food over the surface of the wok or pan, so that everything cooks evenly. I prefer to use one of the new heat-resistant silicone spatulas such as the ones made by Le Creuset, which can resist temperatures up to 650°F (345°C).

TASTING
Don't forget to taste the dish before you put it on the serving plate. Many recipes call for salt and pepper to taste. This is the time to adjust the season-

ing. I always save the sesame oil until the end, since its flavor tends to evaporate in high heat.

WATER BLANCHING

This technique softens vegetables while preserving their vibrant colors. It is commonly used for firmer vegetables, such as broccoli and carrots. Place the vegetable into boiling water for several minutes. Drain and rinse under cold water to stop the cooking process. In most cases, blanching food precedes stir-frying, which completes the cooking process. Blanched foods can also be served with sauces or used as garnishes.

Ingredients

My pantry and refrigerator are my treasure boxes. I go to these boxes when I am happy and hungry, when I am social and creative. With the following "treasures" on hand, a healthy and delicious meal is just minutes away.

My home is one hour from the nearest Asian market districts. Yet thanks to an explosion of interest in healthy foods, and Asian foods in particular, I don't have to travel that far. I can now easily find my ingredients in the Asian sections of my local health food stores and supermarkets.

BABY BOK CHOY

Baby bok choy has dark green leaves and a thick white stem about 6 to 8 inches long. It is a smaller, younger version of bok choy that tastes sweeter and is less fibrous.

BAMBOO SHOOTS

These come from the tips of bamboo stalks. The crisp, pale flesh has a mild flavor. Rinse canned or bottled shoots in cold water before using. Look for shredded shoots to save time. If you are lucky enough to find fresh shoots, be sure to give them a try. Wash, peel, and blanch the shoots in boiling water for 10 minutes before cooking.

CANOLA OIL

I prefer using canola oil for most types of cooking. Rich in monounsaturated fats and low in saturated fats, it also contains a good amount of linolenic acid, an essential omega-3 fat. With its mild, bland taste it is an all-purpose cooking oil that doesn't interfere with flavors. You can substitute vegetable oil, corn oil, soybean, or sunflower oil for canola oil.

CHILI GARLIC PASTE

Made from red or green chilies, garlic, salt and other seasonings, it is sold in jars. Look for varieties that are low in sodium. Refrigerate after opening.

CHILI PEPPERS

There is a wide variety of chilies to choose from. You can choose and substitute among chilies based on your passion for spicy food. Choose fresh chilies without brown patches or black spots.

After handling chilies, don't touch your eyes, lips, or other sensitive areas. Wash your hands, knives, and cutting board thoroughly with soapy water. You may want to wear gloves when you prepare very hot chilies. In this book I use the following types:

Jalapeño (medium hot): This cone-shaped pepper is usually a shiny green and turns red when ripe. It is the standard barometer for spiciness among chilies.

Fresno (hot): This California-grown chili resembles the jalapeño but is slightly broader—about 2 inches long and 1 inch wide.

Serrano (very hot): Slender and much hotter than jalapeño, it comes in green, red, and yellow. It also comes dried, about 1 inch long.

CILANTRO

Also called Chinese parsley, it has a uniquely fragrant, slightly musky flavor and is a flavorful addition to a variety of dishes.

COCONUT MILK

Coconut milk is high in fat and sometimes difficult to find. Substitute coconut juice or coconut powder, or dilute it by half with soymilk. Always look for reduced-fat brands.

CURRY

Curry comes in powder and paste forms. Curry powder is a combination of ground spices, including cumin, coriander, turmeric, cinnamon, and more. Curry paste has a range of flavors and different levels of spiciness. All of them contain curry spices and oil. Red curry contains red chilies while green curry contains green chilies. Yellow curry contains a blend of dried spices. Try them all and find the types that fit your taste. I prefer curry powder because I can better control the amount of oil and spices in the dish. Curry has a very strong flavor, so a little can make a big impression.

DONG QUAI

Also known as angelica, it is sold in three forms—knobs, slices, and pills. Knobs have an ivory color with brown veins and are usually 1 inch long and 3 inches in diameter. Like ginseng roots, they require a long cooking time. Knobs weigh about 1 ounce each. When refrigerated in an airtight jar, *dong quai* can last 8 to 12 months. Slices are about ⅛ inch thick and 3 or 4 inches in diameter. Stored in an airtight jar in the refrigerator, they can last 8 to 12 months.

DRIED BLACK DATES

Black dates look a bit like prunes and have a smoky fragrance. They are about ¾ inch long and ½ inch in diameter with a small pit inside. Available in Asian supermarkets and herb shops, they are often used with *dong quai* and ginseng. Dates are good for PMS and regulating menopause symptoms.

EDAMAME (FRESH GREEN SOYBEANS)

These soybeans are harvested when the beans are still green and sweet. They are high in protein and fiber. Edamame is found in health food stores and Asian markets, shelled or still in the pod.

To serve edamame as a snack, boil in lightly salted water for 15 to 20 minutes. Shelled edamame can be cooked with other ingredients for a vegetarian main dish.

FISH SAUCE

This thin, clear brown sauce is made from fermented shrimp or fish and has a very fishy odor and salty taste. Don't let the smell stop you from trying it. The odor greatly diminishes after cooking. It is popular throughout Southeast Asia and southern China. It is sold in bottles in the Asian section of supermarkets, health-food stores, and Asian specialty markets. It will keep for several months without refrigeration.

GRAPE LEAVES

These come from grapevines. The easy way to get fresh ones is from your own grapevine. You can also find them frozen in many stores. Substitute grape leaves for banana leaves, which you can find at some florist greenhouses and at Asian markets.

GYOZA SKINS

These are similar to wonton wrappers, only slightly thicker. They can be found in the produce section of your supermarket near the tofu.

HONEY

Produced by bees from the nectar of flowers, it is a great alternative to sugar. There are many varieties of honey, which range in color from white to dark brown. The lighter the color, the milder the flavor.

Raw honey contains protective compounds, which kill bacteria, disinfect cuts, and help wounds heal faster. Next time you get a small cut or scrape, try a little honey.

LEEKS

This member of the onion family with white bulbs and long-bladed green leaves has a sweeter and less pungent taste than regular onions. Leeks are often very muddy or sandy, so it is important to clean them well. First slice off and discard the root end and tough outer green leaves. Then split the bulb lengthwise, separating the layers of the bulb and leaves. Soak them in cold water for 5 minutes, then gently remove the stubborn grit with a brush under running water.

LEMONGRASS

This herb has a delicate lemon aroma and flavor. Fresh lemongrass has a 3-foot-long green stalk and a 5- to 7-inch bulblike base. Use only the base. Peel and discard the external tough, dry leaves. Shredded bulbs are used to flavor soup while minced bulbs are used in sauces. Use lemon peel as a substitute. You can find lemongrass in the produce department of some supermarkets.

MEAT ALTERNATIVES (MEAT ANALOGS)

There are many meat alternatives on the market. They contain soy protein or tofu and other ingredients mixed together to simulate various kinds of meat. These meat alternatives are sold refrigerated, frozen, canned, or dried. Usually they can be used the same way as the foods they replace.

MISO

Miso is a rich, salty smooth paste that characterizes the essence of Asian cooking, especially in Japan. It is made from soybeans and a grain such as rice, plus salt and a mold culture, and then aged in cedar vats for one to three years. Miso can be used to flavor a variety of foods, such as soups, sauces, dressings, and marinades. Store miso in the refrigerator, where it will keep for several months.

MUSHROOMS

Mushrooms are a great, simple way to add flavor to your cooking. Their delicate flavors go well with ginseng. Thanks to the extraordinary variety of foods available today, you can now find many kinds of fresh mushrooms in stores, but feel free to substitute one for another. Most mushrooms are available in plastic packages or in bulk. For fresh mushrooms, look for firm, dry flesh free of blemishes. Buy them as you need them, since they tend to become slimy when stored too long in the refrigerator. If you have to put them in the refrigerator, it is best to place them in a paper bag or wrap them in paper towels. In this book I use the following mushrooms.

Shiitake: See pages 25 to 28.

Oyster: This shell-shaped mushroom has a mild, delicate flavor. Discard the knobby stem and wash the caps before using.

Enoki: This cream-colored, long-stemmed, small-capped mushroom has a delicate flavor.

NOODLES

This book calls for the following noodles, but you can substitute them for each other. Always soak dry bean and rice noodles before cooking, but not wheat noodles. Use angel hair or linguine as a substitute for thin bean and rice noodles; use fettuccine to substitute for wide rice noodles.

Bean Threads: These fine white noodles are made from ground mung beans and come in various lengths and thicknesses. They are sold in neat bundles in plastic packages. They will keep in a dry, tightly sealed container for up to 6 months. They are popular in soups, cold noodle dishes, and fillings.

Rice Noodles: Made from long-grain rice flour, these white noodles come in a variety of shapes and thicknesses. Refrigerate fresh ones and cook within a couple of days. Keep the dry form in a tightly sealed container in a dry and cool place for up to 6 months. Rice noodles are popular in stir-fried foods, cold noodle dishes, and soups.

Soba Noodles: Made from a blend of buckwheat and wheat flours, these Japanese noodles also come in flavored varieties, including green tea, vegetable, or wild yam. They can be found in health-food and Asian food stores.

Udon Noodles: These are Japanese noodles made with wheat flour and water. They are ideal for soup and stir-fried dishes.

Wheat Noodles: These are made from white flour and water. Sometimes eggs are added. They are sold fresh or dry and come in various shapes.

OLIVE OIL

Rich in monounsaturated fats and low in saturated fats, olive oil comes in several varieties, from rich-tasting extra-virgin oil from the first pressing to the solvent-extracted oil that is bland in taste and used for general cooking. Use extra-virgin oil when the taste of the oil is important, such as in some salad dressing. Some olive oil is labeled "light," meaning it is light in taste, not calories.

RICE

Long-grain: It consists of long slender grains, about four times as long as they are wide. It's the favored rice in China. When cooked, the rice separates easily and is less starchy than short grain. It is perfect for making fried rice dishes.

Short-grain: These are plump oval grains, which are preferred in the eastern parts of Asia. High in starch, the rice sticks together when cooked. It is used as an accompaniment to main dishes, and for Japanese sushi and Chinese congee (a rice soup).

Glutinous: Also know as sweet or sticky rice, it is a variety of short-grain, with a short, round, pearl-like form. High in starch, it turns translucent when cooked, as well as soft and sticky. It is widely used in Asian festival dishes and desserts.

Sweet Rice Flour: This is made with glutinous rice and is widely used in Asian desserts. It is much stickier than rice flour made from long-grain rice. Asian and some health food stores carry it in small plastic packages.

Wild Rice: Not really rice at all, it is a seed of an aquatic grass that grows wild in the Great Lakes area. It's low in fat, high in B vitamins, and rich in protein. Wild rice has a chewy texture and nutty flavor.

RICE VINEGAR

Made from rice, it has a less acidic taste than cider or wine vinegar. It comes in black, red, and yellow. Black vinegar is dark in color and strong in taste; red vinegar is sweet and spicy; yellow is very mild. There are various seasoned rice vinegars available on the market, such as garlic, basil, and chili pepper. You can substitute cider vinegar for any of them.

RICE WINE

Made with glutinous rice, yeast, and spring water, it has a rich, sweetish mellow taste. Dry sherry can be substituted, but not grape wines.

RICE WRAPPERS

These thin, translucent sheets are made with rice and water. They are the Southeast Asian version of the tortilla, used for wrapping various fillings. Before using, briefly soak in warm water till soft. Store in a dry and cool place for up to 6 months.

ROCK SUGAR

This amber-color crystallized sugar comes in big or small chunks. To break the large pieces, wrap in a kitchen towel, place on a hard surface, and break them with a hammer. Rock sugar is available in Asian grocery stores, sold in plastic bags. Stored in an airtight glass jar in dry and cool place, it will last up to 12 months.

SEAWEED

Also called kelp, it is a nutritious sea vegetable that is a good source of iron and iodine. It has an olive-brown color and comes in threads, sheets, strips, and granules. Some varieties are dry and must be soaked in warm water and softened before using. Other varieties have been roasted and seasoned and require no presoaking. The recipes in this book call for roasted seaweed. Store dry kelp in a sealed container in your pantry for up to 6 months.

Nori is a type of seaweed that is usually toasted or dried. It's used as a wrapper, garnish, or soup flavoring. It comes in sheets, strips, or crumbled. It's available in Asian markets or health-food stores.

SESAME OIL

It is made from toasted sesame seeds and has a strong nutty flavor and aroma. It is so flavorful that a small amount will add a distinctive taste to dishes. The darker the oil, the stronger the flavor. Since it heats rapidly and the flavor evaporates easily, add it to the dish at the end of cooking, or use it in a sauce, but do not use it as cooking oil. It is sold in bottles and is best stored in a cool dark place. Don't refrigerate; it will turn cloudy.

SESAME SHAKERS, OR GOMASIO

Sesame shakers, from Eden Foods, contain roasted, chopped organic sesame seeds combined with other flavorful ingredients and are packed in jars with shaker tops for easy sprinkling on foods. A little shaken on rice creates a balanced, whole-protein meal. Different varieties contain sea salt, seaweed, and garlic. They are a good substitute in recipes that call for toasted sesame seeds.

SOY CHEESE

Soy cheese is made from soy milk. It comes in many different varieties, including Swiss, Cheddar, Monterey Jack, and mozzarella. Soy cheese makes an easy substitute for regular cheese. Be aware that most soy cheese contains casein, which is derived from cow's milk, so it is not a good substitute for those who cannot tolerate dairy.

SOY CREAMER

A nondairy substitute for coffee creamer, soy creamer contains all of the benefits of soy. It can also be used in desserts.

SOY DESSERTS

Nondairy frozen desserts are made from soy milk or soy yogurt. Soy ice cream is one of the most popular desserts made from soybeans. These desserts contain the nutrients of soy, and most have less fat than frozen dairy desserts.

SOY FLOUR

Soy flour is made from roasted soybeans ground into a fine powder. There are three kinds of soy flour available: natural or full-fat, which contains the natural oils found in the soybean; defatted; and lecithinated, which has additional lecithin, the health-promoting fat found in soy.

All soy flours give a protein boost to recipes. However, defatted soy flour is an even more concentrated source of protein than full-fat soy flour. Although used mainly by the food industry, soy flour can be found in natural-foods stores and some supermarkets. Soy flour is gluten-free, so yeast-raised breads made with soy flour are more dense in texture. Replace about one-fourth of the wheat flour with soy flour in recipes for muffins, cakes, cookies, pancakes, and quick breads. It won't affect the flavor, but it will make baked goods lighter and more nourishing.

SOY MARGARINE AND SOY SHORTENING

Soy margarine and shortening are made from soy oil (see page 60) that has been hydrogenated to make them solid. You can also find reduced-fat margarine, which contains less fat than butter.

SOYMILK OR SOY BEVERAGES

Made from ground soybeans, water, sweetener, and salt, this thick, dairy-free beverage is a great alternative for those who are lactose intolerant, or who want to reduce fat intake and increase the amount of soy in their diet. It comes in different flavors and is easy to use in desserts and beverages. It is sold mostly in aseptic containers (nonrefrigerated and shelf-stable), and in quart or half-gallon containers in the dairy case. In recipes, soymilk can be substituted for cow's milk cup for cup. You can reduce the fat in recipes that call for coconut milk by replacing half the coconut milk with soymilk.

SOY NUT BUTTER

Made from roasted, whole soy nuts, which are then crushed and blended with soy oil and other ingredients, soy nut butter makes a good peanut butter substitute with significantly less fat.

SOY OIL

The most widely used oil in the United States, soy oil is extracted from whole soybeans. The oil sold in grocery stores under the generic name "vegetable oil" is usually 100 percent soy oil or a blend of soy and other oils. Read the label. Soy oil is high in polyunsaturated fat. Soy oil handles high temperatures well. It is good to use for stir-frying or deep-frying.

SOY SAUCE

This is made from fermented soybeans, water, salt, and sometimes wheat. The two main types are light and dark.

Dark soy sauce is matured longer. It is thicker and tastes stronger than light soy sauce. It is used for flavor and for added color in dishes. The light sauce is used in dipping sauces. You can also find low-sodium brands on the market. I like to use naturally fermented soy sauce, which is sold at health-food stores and in the Asian section of some supermarkets. To reduce sodium in regular soy sauce at home, simply replace half of the soy sauce called for in the recipe with lemon juice, rice vinegar, or water. Soy sauce will keep for several months without refrigeration.

Shoyu is soy sauce made from a blend of soybeans and wheat; tamari is made only from soybeans and is a by-product of making miso.

SOY SPROUTS

These crisp sprouts of germinated soybeans are an excellent source of nutrition. They are high in protein and packed with vitamin C. They can be found in Asian markets and health-food stores. Soy sprouts must be cooked quickly at low heat, or they will get mushy. They are also ideal for salads or soups.

SOY YOGURT

Soy yogurt is made from soymilk. Its creamy texture makes it an easy substitute for regular yogurt. It comes in variety of flavors and is available in natural-foods stores. Look for a brand with low sugar content. It works well in smoothies and other desserts.

SYRUPS

Syrups are made from maple, rice, and barley malt. They are less sweet than white sugar, not as overpowering as honey, and some also contain potassium, calcium, iron, and B vitamins.

TEMPEH

A chunky, tender soybean cake, it is traditionally used in Indonesian cooking. Made with fermented soybeans mixed with a variety of grains, such as rice and barley, it has a smoky or nutty flavor. Tempeh can be marinated and grilled and added to soups, casseroles, or chili.

TERIYAKI SAUCE

This is similar to soy sauce, but has additional ingredients, such as pineapple juice, chili pepper, ginger, garlic, or sugar. It has a savory, sweet flavor and works well as a marinade sauce. It is ideal for time-saving cooking. You get several ingredients in one bottle. Refrigerate after opening. I prefer the brand name Kim's, made with natural ingredients. Or make your own (page 90).

TOFU AND TOFU-BASED PRODUCTS

Tofu, also known as soybean curd, is a soft, cheeselike food made by curdling fresh hot soymilk with a coagulant. Tofu is a bland product that easily absorbs the flavors of other ingredients while being cooked. Tofu is rich in high-quality protein and B vitamins and low in sodium.

Fresh tofu comes in three different varieties: extra firm, firm, and soft. Each type also comes as low-fat. You can find them in the refrigerated section of most supermarkets. They are sold as 16-ounce blocks packed in water-filled plastic tubs. Firm tofu is dense and solid. It can be cubed and served in soups, stir-fried, or grilled. Firm tofu is higher in protein, fat, and calcium than other forms of tofu. Soft tofu is good for recipes that call for blending in the tofu.

Silken tofu is not the same as fresh tofu. It is creamy and can be used as a replacement for sour cream in many dip recipes. It comes in a rectangular cardboard container. You don't need to refrigerate it, and it has a long shelf life. It stays fresh until opened. Silken tofu has a custardlike consistency. It works well for salad dressings, desserts, and soups. It comes in soft, firm, and extra-firm and light and low-fat varieties.

Baked seasoned tofu is made by pressing water out of fresh tofu, marinating it in seasonings, and baking. It has a brownish color and resilient texture. It is an ideal meat substitute in stir-fried dishes and tossed into salads. I like the White Wave brand, which comes in four flavors.

WATER CHESTNUTS

The crunchiest of vegetables, this pale, almost translucent tuber is hard to find fresh. In fact, I have never seen them fresh in this country. Canned ones come in 8-ounce cans, soaked in water, with mildly sweet and starchy flesh. Before use, discard the water and rinse the water chestnuts in fresh water.

WATERCRESS

This vegetable comes in dark green bunches about 6 inches long, with green leaves and tender stems. It has a distinct mustard flavor. Like other green-leafed vegetables, it has a cooling effect and is excellent with yang foods.

WONTON WRAPPERS

Made from wheat flour, water, and sometimes eggs, these 3- to 4-inch yellow-ish squares are wrapped in plastic and can be purchased fresh or frozen. They can be stuffed with various fillings, then steamed, fried, or stewed in soup. Store the wrappers in the refrigerator for up to a week, or freeze for up to several months. Keep wrappers in a bag at all times to retain their moisture. When cooking with the wrappers, take out only one at a time. Leave the rest in the bag, covered with a damp cloth to prevent them from drying.

Safe Thawing of Foods

According to the USDA, most bacteria thrive at temperatures between 40°F and 140°F (5°C to 60°C)—the "danger zone" for bacterial growth.

- The best way to thaw meat is to transfer it from the freezer to the refrigerator, where the temperature is high enough for the meat and seafood to thaw and cold enough to prevent bacterial growth.
- For a shorter thawing time, place the frozen item in a tightly sealed plastic bag and leave it in a sink filled with cold water. This will prevent moisture loss from the meat and seafood and contamination from the environment. Change the water frequently.
- Thawing meat and seafood in a microwave oven is not the best method. The exterior of the food will be overcooked before the interior begins to thaw.

Reading Food Labels

There's so much information included on food labels these days—ingredients, nutrition information, dietary recommendations, and more. We're told to read the label to make sure the food we're buying is healthy. Reading the label is of little use, though, if you don't understand what the terms used mean. Let me decipher some of these terms for you.

Amino Acids: Amino acids are essential for human survival and muscle growth. Soy protein can contain all nine of the essential amino acids, and their quality is comparable to that in animal protein.

Antioxidants: These are substances such as vitamins C and E and minerals that prevent the chemical reactions that generate toxic oxygen molecules (often called "free radicals"), which damage the body and contribute to many diseases. Antioxidants help to maintain overall health.

Calcium: This mineral helps build strong bones. The richest source of calcium is dairy products, but soy and many vegetables also contain significant amounts of calcium.

Cholesterol: A soft, waxy substance, it is found among the lipids (fats) in the bloodstream and in all your body's cells. It's an important part of a healthy body because it's used to form cell membranes, some hormones, and other needed tissues. But a high level of cholesterol in the blood—hypercholesterolemia—is a major risk factor for coronary heart disease. Limit yourself to 300 milligrams per day.

Complex Carbohydrates: These come from fruits, vegetables, whole grains, beans, and other legumes. Refined carbohydrates, such as white-flour products, are stripped of many of their most important nutrient components and can quickly become "empty calories."

Fat-Free: The product contains less than 0.5 grams of fat per serving.

Fiber: Dietary fiber is present only in plant foods, such as whole grains, fruits, and vegetables. Though not digested, fiber is essential to good health.

Fiber components act like internal cleansers, helping in the passage of wastes through the body. Low-fat diets rich in fruits and vegetables may reduce the risk of some cancers. There are two basic types of fiber—insoluble and soluble.

Soluble Fiber is contained in oats, beans, and such fruits as apples, bananas, and pears. Oats have a greater proportion of soluble fiber than any other grain. When eaten on a regular basis as part of a low-fat, low-cholesterol diet, soluble fiber has been shown to help lower blood cholesterol.

Insoluble Fiber is in whole grains and other vegetables and fruits. Insoluble fiber is essential to healthy digestion.

Kosher: Food prepared according to a strict set of Jewish dietary laws. The term does not imply any nutritional qualities.

Isoflavones: These are health-promoting chemicals found in high levels in soybeans (see page 23).

Light/Lite: This means the product contains 50 percent less fat than the regular product.

Low-Fat: Generally, *low-fat* means the product has no more than 3 grams of fat per serving.

Organic: These are foods grown or produced with little or no synthetic fertilizers or pesticides.

Pareve/Parve: This is one category in kosher dietary laws; food has neither meat nor dairy ingredients.

Preservatives: These are substances added to food to protect against decay, spoilage, or fermentation.

Reduced Fat or Less Fat: Labels products that contain at least 25 percent less fat (in grams) or calories than the regular product.

Reduced Sodium: The product contains at least 25 percent less sodium than the regular product. Limit yourself to 2,400 milligrams per day.

Serving Size: It is different from what we normally think it is; it is usually smaller. Be sure to check the package for the standard serving size.

Whole Foods: This characterizes unrefined or unprocessed foods, such as whole grains, that retain all of their nutritional value.

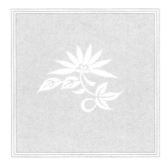

3. Stocks, Sauces, and Condiments

To this day in some rural Asian communities, the matchmaker still plays a significant role in bringing young men and women together. Matchmakers busily travel between the homes of eligible young people, trying to arrange marriages. My grandparents were married through an introduction by a matchmaker.

When my grandmother made stocks and sauces she always said, "Let's do some matchmaking today." She had many freshly chopped spices and other ingredients set around the table with several empty jars nearby. Throwing in a little bit of this and that into the jars, she soon made various sauces and stocks. Grandmother told me, "The key is to match the ones you think will get along." By this she meant one should balance the yin (female) ingredients with yang (male) ingredients to make a good match.

Depending on the season and what ingredients she had on hand, Grandmother never made the same sauce twice, yet they all tasted superior. I made my sauces my grandmother's way for years. Then I realized that this spontaneous approach is foreign to my students and friends, and difficult to master. I started to make notes and keep a record of my experiments. All the sauces in this book are based on this process. Use these recipes as a starting point for your own. Perhaps your sauces will reflect your idea of a good marriage. Is the chili too hot-tempered for you? Take it out! With practice I am sure you too will enjoy matchmaking.

Before you begin, have plenty of small containers available. You can get them in the supermarket salad section or at cookware stores. Double or triple recipes you like. Most of the sauces can be made ahead and stored in a tightly sealed container in the refrigerator. Be sure to use a clean, dry spoon each time you serve the sauce.

A rich stock or broth is the foundation of a delicious soup. Fortunately, to make a broth you only need good water and a few fresh ingredients you probably have on hand. Simmer for 40 to 60 minutes.

Use the following stocks as the base for soups and cooking sauces. If you want a light sauce, strain and pour into a tightly sealed container, and eat the remaining solids over rice or noodles. If you like a thick sauce then place the stock in a blender and blend until smooth. Allow the stock to cool before using. The vegetable solids left over from stock can be composted.

For fast and delicious cooking, sauces and broth are a must. Make them ahead and keep them in your freezer and refrigerator. Refrigerated, the stock will keep for three or four days. Frozen, it will keep for several weeks. If you are cooking for one or two people, you can make less by simply cutting the ingredients in half.

Recipes throughout this book call for different stocks and sauces. If you don't have a particular one on hand and are pressed for time, don't let it stop you from making a delicious meal. Mix and match your own, or even use purchased stocks and sauces as a base and add your favorite fresh ingredients.

Some recipes in this section call for fresh whole ginseng. If you don't have it, substitute dry whole ginseng, sliced ginseng, or even ginseng tea bags.

Ginseng-Chicken Stock

Many chicken stock recipes call for chicken bones or the whole chicken, which requires 4 or 5 hours to cook and is high in fat. I have come up with this healthy and simple way to make chicken stock. People who have tasted it tell me that after trying this homemade stock they never want to use any other kind. It is well worth your time and effort. This stock has less fat and takes less time than traditional recipes, yet it is much more flavorful than the commercial brands.

2 TABLESPOONS CANOLA OIL

2 TABLESPOONS ¼-INCH FRESH GINGER CHUNKS

6 CLOVES GARLIC, MINCED

1 MEDIUM ONION, CHOPPED

1 POUND BONELESS, SKINLESS CHICKEN BREASTS,
    CUT INTO 1-INCH CHUNKS

3 CUPS SPRING WATER

6 CUPS CANNED LOW-SODIUM, LOW-FAT CHICKEN BROTH

2 TO 3 WHOLE FRESH GINSENG ROOTS (ABOUT 1 OUNCE)

3 CUPS FRESH OR FROZEN CORN KERNELS

SALT AND WHITE PEPPER TO TASTE

Heat a nonstick wok or skillet over medium heat and coat it with the oil. Sauté the ginger, garlic, and onion until fragrant, 1 to 2 minutes. Add the chicken and sauté until the chicken browns slightly, 2 to 3 minutes.

In a large pot, bring the water and chicken broth to a boil. Add the chicken mixture, ginseng, and corn. Bring to a second boil. Reduce the heat and simmer for 50 to 60 minutes. Season with salt and pepper.

Strain the liquid through a colander, pressing out as much liquid as possible. Let cool. Pour stock into a container and refrigerate or freeze.

Makes 5 1/2 cups

> **TIP**
>
> FOR A FAST, THAI-FLAVORED CHICKEN SIDE DISH, PLACE THE CHICKEN AND SOLIDS IN A BOWL, ADD 2 TABLESPOONS COCONUT MILK, 2 TABLESPOONS CILANTRO LEAVES, AND 1 MINCED RED CHILI PEPPER. MIX THOROUGHLY. SERVE OVER NOODLES, RICE, OR AS THE FILLING FOR FRESH SPRING ROLLS (PAGE 122).

Spicy Vegetable Stock

You may be surprised at how flavorful this spicy stock is. The fresh vegetables blend together to form a rich base for many soups and sauces. Adjust the amount of chili pepper based on your preferences. Use this recipe as a basic recipe; you can vary according to the vegetables available in your garden or that are in season.

3 TABLESPOONS CANOLA OIL

1 CUP FRESH MINCED SHIITAKE OR OYSTER MUSHROOMS

2 CHILI PEPPERS, MINCED

2 CELERY STALKS, CHOPPED

2 MEDIUM CARROTS, PEELED AND CUT DIAGONALLY INTO ¼-INCH CHUNKS

1 CUP CHOPPED CHINESE CABBAGE

1 CUP SUNFLOWER SPROUTS

¼ CUP CHOPPED CHIVES

6 CUPS SPRING WATER

2 TO 3 WHOLE FRESH GINSENG ROOTS (ABOUT 1 OUNCE, OPTIONAL)

3 TABLESPOONS CILANTRO LEAVES

2 TEASPOONS SESAME OIL

SALT AND WHITE PEPPER TO TASTE

Heat a nonstick wok or skillet over medium heat and coat it with the oil. Add the mushrooms, chilies, and celery and sauté for 1 minute. Add the carrots, cabbage, sprouts, and chives. Cover and cook, stirring occasionally, until carrots soften, about 2 minutes.

Add the water and ginseng, and bring to a boil. Reduce the heat and simmer for 45 minutes. Add the sesame oil. Season with salt and pepper.

Strain the liquid through a colander, pressing out as much liquid as possible. Let cool. Pour stock into a container and refrigerate or freeze. Eat the ginseng, if desired; it has a very strong flavor. Discard or compost the solids.

Makes 5 cups

MATCHMAKING

LIKE I SAID IN THE INTRODUCTION TO THIS CHAPTER, MY GRANDMOTHER WOULD SAY THAT MAKING STOCKS AND SAUCES IS LIKE MATCHMAKING. IN ASIA, MANY MARRIAGES WERE ARRANGED BY MATCHMAKERS. THE MATCHMAKERS FOUND A SUITABLE FAMILY AND SET UP THE FIRST MEETING FOR THE YOUNG COUPLE AND THEIR FAMILIES. TEA WAS ALWAYS SERVED BY THE PROSPECTIVE BRIDE. AT THE MEETING THE THE MOTHER OF THE PROSPECTIVE GROOM EXAMINED THE YOUNG WOMAN CLOSELY. IF SHE DRANK THE TEA BEFORE THE LEAVES SANK TO THE BOTTOM, SHE WAS CONSIDERED IMPATIENT. THE MARRIAGE VERY LIKELY WOULD NOT OCCUR BETWEEN THE YOUNG COUPLE. IF INSTEAD SHE COULD WAIT UNTIL THE HOT WATER UNFURLED THE TEA LEAVES AND THEY SANK TO THE BOTTOM OF THE TEACUP, SHE WOULD BE APPROVED FOR HER GOOD MANNERS.

LUCKILY, MY AMERICAN MOTHER-IN-LAW SERVED ME TEA MADE WITH TEA BAGS THE FIRST TIME WE MET.

Vegetable and Mushroom Stock

Although you can buy a variety of vegetable stocks in the supermarket, there is nothing quite like a homemade mushroom stock for enhancing the flavor of soup and stews. It takes only a little effort and can cook while you prepare other dishes in the kitchen, do housework, or read a magazine. Use only the freshest vegetables for this stock.

3 TABLESPOONS CANOLA OIL

1 TABLESPOON CHOPPED FRESH GINGER

3 CLOVES GARLIC, MINCED

1½ CUPS FRESH SHIITAKE OR OYSTER MUSHROOMS,
    CUT INTO SMALL CUBES

1 CUP CHOPPED LEEKS (WHITE PARTS ONLY)

1 CUP SNOW PEAS

6 CUPS SPRING WATER

3 MEDIUM TOMATOES, CHOPPED

3 CUPS FRESH OR FROZEN CORN KERNELS

2 TEASPOONS SESAME OIL

SALT AND BLACK PEPPER TO TASTE

Heat a nonstick wok or skillet over medium heat and coat it with oil. Add the ginger, garlic, mushrooms, and leeks and sauté until the mushrooms are lightly browned, about 1 minute. Add the snow peas and sauté until softened, about 2 minutes.

Add the water, tomatoes, and corn. Bring to a boil. Reduce the heat and simmer for 45 minutes. Stir in the sesame oil. Season with salt and pepper.

Strain the liquid through a colander, pressing out as much liquid as possible. Let cool. Pour stock into a container and refrigerate or freeze. Eat the ginger if desired; it has a very strong flavor. Discard or compost the solids.

Makes 5 cups

Green Tea–Seafood Stock

Traditionally, seafood stock calls for fish heads and bones, which require hours of cooking. I have developed this simple and healthy seafood stock, which I use frequently in the summertime for many of my favorite dishes.

6 GREEN TEA BAGS

8 CUPS BOILING WATER

2 TABLESPOONS CANOLA OIL

2 TABLESPOONS ¼-INCH FRESH GINGER CHUNKS

4 CLOVES GARLIC, QUARTERED

1 CUP MINCED OYSTER OR SHIITAKE MUSHROOMS

1 FRESH RED CHILI PEPPER, MINCED

2 MEDIUM LEEKS (WHITE PARTS ONLY),
    CUT DIAGONALLY INTO ½-INCH CHUNKS

½ POUND SCALLOPS

½ POUND FRESH OR FROZEN WHITE FISH FILLET,
    CUT INTO 2-INCH PIECES

12 SPRIGS CILANTRO

1 TEASPOON WHITE PEPPER

Place the green tea bags in a large pot. Add the boiling water and simmer over low heat for 3 minutes. Use a spoon to press the tea out of the tea bags. Discard the tea bags.

Heat a nonstick wok or skillet over medium heat and coat it with the oil. Add the ginger, garlic, mushrooms, chili, and leeks and sauté until the leeks soften and become fragrant, about 2 minutes.

Add the vegetable mixture to the tea and bring the mixture to a boil. Add the scallops, fish, and cilantro. Return to a boil. Reduce the heat and simmer, uncovered, for 40 minutes. Season with pepper.

Strain the liquid through a colander, pressing out as much liquid as possible. Let cool. Pour stock into a container and refrigerate or freeze.

Makes 4 1/2 cups

Ginseng-Seafood Stock

This ginseng stock is good for the winter months. It is a variation of Green Tea-Seafood Stock (page 75), which is good for the summer.

3 TABLESPOONS CANOLA OIL

1 ½ TABLESPOONS 1-INCH FRESH GINGER CHUNKS

2 LEMONGRASS STALKS, BOTTOM 5 INCHES ONLY (SEE PAGE 54)

1 CUP ½-INCH LEEK CHUNKS (WHITE PART ONLY)

1 CUP OYSTER OR SHIITAKE MUSHROOMS, MINCED

8 CUPS SPRING WATER

2 TO 3 WHOLE FRESH GINSENG ROOTS (ABOUT 1 OUNCE)

½ POUND LARGE SCALLOPS

½ POUND SHELLED RAW SHRIMP WITH TAILS ON

6 SPRIGS WATERCRESS, CUT INTO 2-INCH LENGTHS

SALT AND WHITE PEPPER TO TASTE

Heat a nonstick wok or skillet over medium heat and coat it with the oil. Add the ginger, lemongrass, leeks, and mushrooms and sauté until the leeks soften and become fragrant, about 2 minutes.

Add the water to a big pot and bring to a boil. Add the ginseng, scallops, shrimp, and watercress. Bring to a second boil. Reduce the heat and simmer for 45 minutes.

Strain the liquid through a colander, pressing out as much liquid as possible. Let cool. Pour stock into a container and refrigerate or freeze. Enjoy the solids as a side dish or over rice. Discard the ginger and lemongrass.

Makes 7 ⅓ cups

Spicy Sesame Sauce

This is a good dipping sauce for Fresh Spring Rolls (page 122), or to use as a stir-fry or marinade sauce.

1 TEASPOON WHITE SESAME SEEDS, TOASTED (SEE TIP, PAGE 200)

2 CLOVES GARLIC, MINCED

1 GREEN ONION (GREEN AND WHITE PARTS), FINELY SLICED

1 TEASPOON MINCED FRESH GINGER

¼ CUP TERIYAKI SAUCE (PAGE 90) OR PURCHASED

2 TABLESPOONS FRESH LEMON JUICE

1 TEASPOON SESAME OIL

1 TEASPOON THINLY SHREDDED FRESH RED CHILI PEPPER

Place all the ingredients in a bowl and mix to combine. Cover and let the flavors blend in the refrigerator for about 30 minutes before using.

Makes ¾ cup

Ginger and Garlic Sauce

Dumplings or spring rolls would not be complete without a dipping sauce. This truly superb sauce owes its vibrant flavor to freshly minced ginger and garlic.

1 TEASPOON CANOLA OIL

2 TEASPOONS LOOSE GREEN TEA

½ TABLESPOON MINCED FRESH GINGER

2 CLOVES GARLIC, MINCED

1 GREEN ONION (GREEN PART ONLY), MINCED

3 TABLESPOONS LOW-SODIUM SOY SAUCE

2 TABLESPOONS SOYMILK

2 TABLESPOONS FRESH LEMON JUICE

2 TABLESPOONS RICE VINEGAR

1 TEASPOON SESAME OIL

In a small saucepan, heat the canola oil. Add the green tea leaves and cook, stirring, until the tea is fragrant and crispy, 10 to 20 seconds.

Combine the remaining ingredients in a small bowl. Stir in the green tea and oil. Cover and let the flavors blend in the refrigerator for 30 minutes or up to 1 week.

Makes ½ cup

Spicy Cilantro Sauce

This sauce is full of fire/yang; balance it with vegetables, tofu, or seafood. Use as a stir-fry sauce, or as a marinade.

4 TEASPOONS FRESH LIME JUICE

¼ CUP CHOPPED FRESH CILANTRO

4 MEDIUM CLOVES GARLIC, CHOPPED

2 MEDIUM GREEN ONIONS (GREEN AND WHITE PARTS), CHOPPED

4 SMALL HOT GREEN CHILI PEPPERS, SEEDED AND CHOPPED

2 TEASPOONS GROUND GINGER

½ TEASPOON FRESHLY GROUND WHITE PEPPER

2 TABLESPOONS CANOLA OIL

1 TABLESPOON FISH SAUCE (SEE PAGE 53)

1 TEASPOON HONEY

Place all the ingredients in a blender. Process into a coarse paste. Use immediately or store in a tightly sealed container in the refrigerator for up to 1 week.

Makes ⅔ cup

Savory Oil

This is good for stir-fry and noodle dishes, or as a garnish. Mince the chili peppers with the seeds if you want a spicier sauce.

1 TEASPOON PLUS ¼ CUP CANOLA OIL

2 TEASPOONS LOOSE GREEN TEA

5 CLOVES GARLIC, MINCED

1 TABLESPOON FRESH GINGER, MINCED

2 FRESH RED CHILI PEPPERS, MINCED

2 GREEN ONIONS (WHITE PART ONLY), MINCED

½ TEASPOON SALT

In a small saucepan, heat the 1 teaspoon oil. Add the green tea and cook, stirring, until the tea is fragrant and crispy, about 1 minute.

Place the tea, garlic, ginger, chili, onions, and salt in a short wide-mouth canning jar and mix to combine.

In the same saucepan, heat the ¼ cup oil until it is very hot. Carefully pour the hot oil over the contents of the jar. Partially cover the jar and let cool. Seal the jar tightly and store in the refrigerator for up to 2 weeks. Stir the sauce before using.

Makes ½ cup

TIPS

WEAR RUBBER GLOVES WHEN MINCING CHILI PEPPERS. TURN THE KITCHEN FAN ON BEFORE POURING THE OIL OVER THE CHILI MIXTURE.

East Meets West Sauce

This invention was created after one of my summer parties. This unique dressing tastes great on salad.

¼ CUP SOYMILK

2 TABLESPOONS RICE VINEGAR

½ TABLESPOON OLIVE OIL

2 TEASPOONS FISH SAUCE

2 SMALL CLOVES GARLIC, MINCED

1 TEASPOON MINCED FRESH GINGER

1 GREEN ONION (GREEN PART ONLY), MINCED

Mix all the ingredients in a small container. Use immediately or cover and store in the refrigerator for up to 1 day.

Makes ½ cup

Spicy Lemon–Basil Sauce

This is good for a salad dressing, as a dipping sauce, and for stir-frying. Chop the chili peppers with the seeds if you want a spicier sauce.

¼ CUP PLAIN RICE MILK OR SOYMILK

1 TABLESPOON HONEY

2 TABLESPOONS FRESH LEMON JUICE

2 TABLESPOONS OLIVE OIL

½ CUP BASIL LEAVES, CHOPPED

2 CLOVES GARLIC, CHOPPED

1 SMALL JALAPEÑO CHILI PEPPER, CHOPPED

¼ TEASPOON SALT

¼ TEASPOON WHITE PEPPER

Combine all the ingredients in a blender and process until puréed. Pour into a container and use immediately or cover and store in the refrigerator for up to 2 weeks.

Makes 1 cup

Curry Peanut Sauce

This spicy sweet and sour sauce works great with spring rolls or crunchy noodles.

1 TABLESPOON CANOLA OIL

2 CLOVES GARLIC, MINCED

1 TEASPOON GRATED FRESH GINGER

¼ CUP MINCED ONION

½ CUP UNSALTED PEANUT BUTTER

½ CUP RICE MILK OR SOYMILK

½ TABLESPOON FRESH LEMON JUICE

1 TEASPOON CURRY POWDER

In a small saucepan, heat the oil over medium heat. Add the garlic, ginger, and onion and sauté until the onion softens, 4 to 5 minutes.

Add the peanut butter, rice milk, lemon juice, and curry powder. Cook, stirring, until the sauce is hot and the peanut butter melts, 1 to 2 minutes.

Let the sauce cool. Use immediately or store in the refrigerator in a tightly sealed container for up to a week.

Makes about 1½ cups

TIP

FOR A SMOOTHER SAUCE, PROCESS THE SAUCE IN A FOOD PROCESSOR FOR 20 SECONDS BEFORE COOLING.

Ginger-Mushroom Sauce

A seafood dish would not be the same without a sauce. Asian cooks often use a sauce containing ginger and wine when cooking with seafood.

2 TABLESPOONS THINLY SHREDDED FRESH GINGER

¼ CUP FRESH SHIITAKE MUSHROOMS, MINCED

¼ TEASPOON FRESH RED CHILI PEPPER, MINCED

½ SMALL GREEN ONION (GREEN AND WHITE PARTS), MINCED

3 CLOVES GARLIC, MINCED

3 TABLESPOONS RICE WINE

2 TABLESPOONS FRESH LEMON JUICE

2 TABLESPOONS RICE VINEGAR

1 TABLESPOON FISH SAUCE (SEE PAGE 53)

½ TEASPOON SESAME OIL

Mix all the ingredients in a small container. Use immediately, or cover and store in the refrigerator for up to 3 days.

Makes ¾ cup

Yogurt-Mint Sauce

There are many versions of yogurt sauce in India. The three common ingredients in the sauce are yogurt, cucumber, and mint. It's often served with spicy fried and grilled dishes. Here is my interpretation of this classic, sumptuous sauce.

1½ CUPS PLAIN YOGURT

½ CUP CHOPPED, SEEDED, PEELED CUCUMBER

3 TABLESPOONS OLIVE OIL

1 TEASPOON SUGAR

1 CHILI PEPPER, SEEDED AND CHOPPED

1 TEASPOON MINCED FRESH GINGER

1 TABLESPOON FRESH LEMON JUICE

2 TABLESPOONS CHOPPED FRESH MINT LEAVES

SALT TO TASTE

Place all the ingredients in a blender. Purée until smooth. Store in the refrigerator for up to 3 days.

Makes 2 cups

White Wine Sauce

This sauce is good for marinating whole chicken or fish, or on salads that accompany meat and seafood.

1 CUP DRY WHITE WINE

2 TABLESPOONS HONEY

½ CUP REDUCED-FAT MILK OR LIGHT CREAM

¼ CUP OLIVE OIL

1 SMALL ONION, MINCED

2 TABLESPOONS FRESHLY GRATED ORANGE PEEL

1 TABLESPOON CHOPPED FRESH CILANTRO LEAVES

SALT AND BLACK PEPPER TO TASTE

Combine all the ingredients in a glass container. Store in the refrigerator for up to 1 week.

Makes 2 cups

Spicy Ginseng Tea Sauce

Use American ginseng for this recipe. The ginseng's yin will balance the yang of the hot chili pepper.

½ CUP BREWED GINSENG TEA (SEE PAGE 35)

3 TABLESPOONS HONEY

¼ CUP FRESH LIME JUICE

2 TABLESPOONS OLIVE OIL

½ CUP WATERCRESS LEAVES, CHOPPED

3 CLOVES GARLIC, CHOPPED

2 SMALL JALAPEÑO CHILIES, SEEDED AND CHOPPED

½ TEASPOON SALT

½ TEASPOON WHITE PEPPER

Combine all ingredients in a blender and purée into a sauce for 2 minutes. Place the sauce in a large airtight container and store in the refrigerator for up to 1 week.

Makes 1 cup

VARIATION

IF USING THIS SAUCE WITH SEAFOOD, ADD 1 TABLESPOON MINCED GINGER AND 2 TABLESPOONS COOKING WINE.

Orange and Soy Sauce

This sauce is good for dipping, stir-frying, and marinating. It is particularly good with vegetables and tofu.

1 AMERICAN GINSENG TEA BAG

1 CUP BOILING SPRING WATER

1 CUP FRESHLY SQUEEZED ORANGE JUICE

¼ CUP RICE VINEGAR (SEE PAGE 57)

3 TABLESPOONS SOY SAUCE

2 TABLESPOONS OLIVE OIL

1 TABLESPOON FRESH GINGER, MINCED

1 GREEN ONION (GREEN AND WHITE PARTS), MINCED

2 TEASPOONS CHOPPED WATERCRESS LEAVES

1 TEASPOON CHOPPED FRESH CILANTRO LEAVES

Brew the tea bag in the boiling spring water for 5 minutes. Drink the tea, place the contents of tea bag in a glass jar, and discard the bag.

Add the remaining ingredients to the jar and mix thoroughly. Store in the refrigerator for up to 1 week.

Makes 1 ⅓ cups

Teriyaki Sauce

If you like teriyaki sauces, you will love this recipe. This version is much tastier than the common store brands and contains less sodium.

¾ CUP LOW-SODIUM SOY SAUCE

2 TABLESPOONS RICE WINE OR DRY SHERRY

1 TABLESPOON SESAME OIL

2½ TABLESPOONS MAPLE SYRUP

2 LARGE CLOVES GARLIC, MINCED

1 TABLESPOON MINCED FRESH GINGER

2 GREEN ONIONS (WHITE PART ONLY), MINCED

Mix all ingredients in a glass jar. Store in the refrigerator for up to 1 week.

Makes 1⅓ cups

Thai Sauce

This is a variation of a popular sauce from Thailand. It's good for seasoning soups, flavoring noodle dishes, and as a salad dressing or dipping sauce.

½ CUP BREWED GINSENG TEA (SEE PAGE 35)

¼ CUP REDUCED-FAT, UNSWEETENED COCONUT MILK

1 TABLESPOON SLICED OR POWDERED GINSENG

2 TABLESPOONS FRESH LIME JUICE

½ CUP REDUCED-FAT PEANUT BUTTER

4 CLOVES GARLIC, CHOPPED

1 FRESH RED CHILI PEPPER, CHOPPED

1 TABLESPOON HONEY

1 GREEN ONION (GREEN AND WHITE PARTS), CHOPPED

8 FRESH CILANTRO LEAVES, CHOPPED

2 TABLESPOONS FISH SAUCE, OR TO TASTE

Place all the ingredients in a blender. Purée until smooth. Store in the refrigerator for up to 1 week.

Makes 2 cups

Green Chili Sauce

In many Asian countries, people love spicy food, but they particularly love it in combination with other pungent ingredients such as garlic, vinegar, and fish sauce. This delicious sauce is often served as a salad dressing, or as a dipping sauce.

1 TEASPOON CANOLA OIL

3 FRESH GREEN CHILI PEPPERS, MINCED

2 CLOVES GARLIC, MINCED

½ CUP BREWED GREEN TEA (SEE PAGE 39)

1 TABLESPOON HONEY

¼ CUP RICE VINEGAR

1 TABLESPOON FISH SAUCE (SEE PAGE 53)

Heat a small saucepan over medium-high heat. Add the canola oil. Add the chili and garlic and sauté until fragrant, about 30 seconds. Add the green tea, honey, vinegar, and fish sauce. Bring to a boil.

Let the sauce cool. Use immediately or store in a tightly sealed container in the refrigerator for up to 1 week.

Makes 1 cup

Creamy Basil Sauce

This cooling sauce with basil and tofu makes a great dip for spicy dishes, as well as a great salad dressing for summer.

½ CUP BREWED GINSENG TEA (SEE PAGE 35)

½ CUP SOYMILK

3 CLOVES GARLIC, MINCED

1 CUP FRESH BASIL LEAVES, CHOPPED

6 OUNCES (½ PACKAGE) EXTRA-FIRM SILKEN TOFU

1 TABLESPOON OLIVE OIL

SALT AND BLACK PEPPER TO TASTE

Place all the ingredients in a blender and blend until smooth. Use immediately or store in a tightly sealed container in the refrigerator for up to 3 days.

Makes 2 cups

Spicy Honey-Basil Sauce

This versatile sauce is one of my favorites. I often triple the recipe and have it on hand to use as a dipping sauce or as a salad dressing.

2 TEA BAGS AMERICAN GINSENG TEA

1 CUP BOILING SPRING WATER

2 TABLESPOONS PINE NUTS, TOASTED (SEE TIP, PAGE 96)

1 TABLESPOON HONEY

2 TABLESPOONS FRESH LEMON JUICE

2 TABLESPOONS OLIVE OIL

½ CUP PACKED FRESH BASIL LEAVES

2 CLOVES GARLIC, MINCED

1 SMALL FRESH OR DRY RED CHILI PEPPER OR 1 MEDIUM JALAPEÑO
   CHILI, CHOPPED (INCLUDE THE SEEDS IF YOU LIKE IT SPICY)

¼ TEASPOON SALT

¼ TEASPOON GROUND WHITE PEPPER

Brew the tea bag in the boiling spring water for 5 minutes. Place the contents of tea bag and the tea in a blender, and discard the bag.

Add the remaining ingredients to the blender and process until puréed. Use immediately or store in a tightly sealed container in the refrigerator for up to 1 week.

Makes 1 cup

All-Occasion Sauce

I have used this pungent sauce for turkey, chicken, tofu, and fish. If you are cooking a larger turkey, double or triple the recipe.

¼ CUP EXTRA-VIRGIN OLIVE OIL

¼ CUP BREWED GINSENG TEA (SEE PAGE 35)
     OR GREEN TEA (SEE PAGE 39)

2 TABLESPOONS FRESH LEMON JUICE

6 CLOVES GARLIC, MINCED

1 TEASPOON MINCED FRESH GINGER

3 TABLESPOONS MINCED CHIVES

1 TEASPOON MINCED FRESH SERRANO
     OR OTHER CHILI PEPPER (OPTIONAL)

⅛ TEASPOON SALT

Place all the ingredients in a glass jar. Store in the refrigerator and let flavors meld for at least 2 hours. It will taste best if stored in the refrigerator for 2 days (store refrigerated up to 5 days) before using, to let the fresh seasonings flavor the oil.

Makes 1 cup

Pesto Sauce

I like to make this sauce on weekends and freeze it in individual ice cube trays and transfer it to freezer bags for storage. On weeknights, I simply take out the pesto cubes and use them to flavor vegetables, pasta, shrimp, or sliced chicken breast. In almost no time, I can enjoy a healthy, delicious meal.

1 ¼ CUPS FRESH BASIL LEAVES

2 CLOVES GARLIC, PRESSED

3 TABLESPOONS PINE NUTS, TOASTED (SEE TIP, BELOW)

3 TABLESPOONS OLIVE OIL

1 MEDIUM TOMATO, CHOPPED (ABOUT 1 ¼ CUPS)

1 TEASPOON HONEY

SALT AND BLACK PEPPER TO TASTE

Rinse and drain the basil leaves. Place all the ingredients in a blender or food processor. Puree until smooth. (You may need to stop several times to scrape the ingredients off the side of the blender or food processor with a wooden or rubber spatula.)

Makes 1 cup

TIPS

TO TOAST PINE NUTS OR OTHER NUTS: SPREAD THEM ON A BAKING SHEET AND BAKE IN A 350°F (175°C) OVEN FOR 8 TO 10 MINUTES, OR UNTIL SLIGHTLY BROWN.

TWO EASY WAYS TO STORE THE PESTO SAUCE: SPOON SAUCE INTO AN ICE CUBE TRAY. AFTER THE SAUCE FREEZES, REMOVE THE ICE CUBES AND STORE IN PLASTIC FREEZER BAGS. OR OPEN A SMALL PLASTIC BAG AND PLACE IN A GLASS TO SUPPORT IT. SPOON THE SAUCE INTO THE BAG. TIE EACH BAG OF SAUCE AND STORE THE BAGS IN A LARGER FREEZER BAG. PESTO CAN BE FROZEN FOR UP TO 3 MONTHS.

Pineapple-Ginseng Sauce

If you like sweet and sour flavor, this sauce is for you. I use it for barbecue dishes. It provides a nice contrasting flavor to grilled meat and seafood.

½ CUP FRESH PINEAPPLE CHUNKS

½ CUP BREWED GINSENG TEA (SEE PAGE 35)

¼ CUP RICE VINEGAR

¼ CUP OLIVE OIL

2 CLOVES GARLIC, MINCED

2 TABLESPOONS HONEY

Place all the ingredients in a blender and purée until smooth. Store in a tightly sealed container in the refrigerator for up to 1 week.

Makes 1½ cups

Apple-Orange Sauce

This is a nice accompaniment for chicken and turkey, or use as a salad dressing. After you refrigerate it, the oil in the sauce will solidify. Warm the container in a bowl of warm water, or let stand at room temperature until liquid before using.

1 TABLESPOON FRESHLY GRATED ORANGE PEEL

¼ CUP OLIVE OIL

1 CUP FRESH APPLE CIDER

¼ CUP WHITE VINEGAR

CONTENTS OF 1 GINSENG TEA BAG (OPTIONAL)

4 GREEN ONIONS, (WHITE PART ONLY), MINCED

SALT AND BLACK PEPPER TO TASTE

Sauté the orange peel in the olive oil over medium heat until fragrant. Remove from the heat. Add the cider, vinegar, and ginseng, if using, and bring to a boil. Simmer for 5 minutes. Stir in the green onions and add salt and pepper. Cool and store in a glass jar in the refrigerator for up to 1 week.

Makes 1 cup

Mango-Ginger Salsa

This colorful and versatile salsa can be used as a dip for chips or crackers. I also serve it with all types of grilled dishes. For variation, try substituting papayas and peaches for the mangoes.

1 RIPE LARGE MANGO, PEELED, PITTED, AND DICED INTO ¼-INCH CUBES

1 SMALL RED ONION, MINCED (ABOUT 1 CUP)

1 TABLESPOON FRESH LEMON JUICE

2 TEASPOONS MINCED FRESH GINGER

2 TEASPOONS OLIVE OIL

¼ CUP CHOPPED BASIL LEAVES

SALT AND BLACK PEPPER TO TASTE

1 (12-OUNCE) PACKAGE EXTRA-FIRM SILKEN TOFU

3 TABLESPOONS CANOLA OIL

2 CLOVES GARLIC, MINCED

1 GREEN ONION (GREEN AND WHITE PARTS ONLY), MINCED

In a medium bowl, mix together all the ingredients. Cover and refrigerate for up to 2 or 3 days.

Makes 2½ cups

Roasted Pepper–Sun-Dried Tomatoes Sauce

My family loves sun-dried tomatoes. After I developed this recipe, for weeks we used it for everything. My son even spread this on his sandwiches and used it as a dip for chips.

1 CUP BOTTLED ROASTED RED BELL PEPPERS, DRAINED

¼ CUP (ABOUT 2 OUNCES) DRY-PACK, SUN-DRIED TOMATOES, CHOPPED

2 CLOVES GARLIC, PEELED

3 TABLESPOONS FRESH LEMON JUICE

2 TABLESPOONS BALSAMIC VINEGAR

Place all the ingredients in a blender or food processor, and process until smooth. Pour into a container. Use immediately or cover and store in the refrigerator for up to 1 week.

Makes 1½ cups

Roasted Pepper–Green Tea Sauce

Roasted peppers are relatively rare in Asian cooking. I was delighted at how they blended with green tea and created this delicious, all-purpose condiment.

1 CUP FRESH OR BOTTLED ROASTED RED BELL PEPPERS, DRAINED

½ CUP BREWED GREEN TEA (SEE PAGE 39)

2 TABLESPOONS (ABOUT 1 OUNCE) DRY-PACKED SUN-DRIED TOMATOES, CHOPPED

2 TABLESPOONS RICE VINEGAR (SEE PAGE 57)

2 CLOVES GARLIC, PEELED

1 TABLESPOON OLIVE OIL

½ TEASPOON WHITE PEPPER

Combine all the ingredients in a blender or food processor and process until smooth. Pour into a container. Use immediately or cover and store in the refrigerator for up to 1 week.

Makes 1 ½ cups

Candied Nuts

I have found that homemade candied nuts are very useful as garnish for salads or stir-fry dishes. You can cook them in a big batch, let them cool, and store in an air-tight sealed container. Refrigerate them for up to 1 week.

3 CUPS WATER

2 CUPS WALNUTS OR PECANS

½ CUP CANOLA OIL

1 CUP SUGAR

In a pot, bring the water to a boil. Blanch nuts for 2 minutes; drain. Spread nuts on a flat surface and let them cool. Pat dry.

In a nonstick cooking pan, heat the oil over medium heat. Stir in the sugar. Reduce heat to low, and cook, stirring constantly, until sugar starts to melt. Stir in the nuts, and cook, stirring, until sugar coats all the nuts.

Spread nuts on paper towels to absorb any excess oil.

Makes about 2 cups

4. Magical Wrappers and Fantastic Finger Foods

My passion for wraps started when I was four years old. My grandmother had just given me a new pair of small red training chopsticks, tied together with a rubber band. The noodles kept slipping from my chopsticks again and again. Finally, I rolled up my sleeves, grabbed the noodles, and stuffed them into my mouth.

Eating with my hands—something that comes naturally to those of us who grew up using chopsticks—is one of my favorite ways of enjoying food. After the episode with the noodles, I found out that there were all kinds of finger foods in wrappers, especially egg rolls, dumplings, mu shu pork, and dim sum. I didn't have to struggle with my little chopsticks, and it was a more efficient way of eating.

After I had a chance to experience other cuisines, I was delighted to find out that there are hundreds of dishes wrapped in various skins, ranging from barbecued chicken and pork, plump shrimp, flavored rice, or fresh vegetables to delicate bean noodles and spicy fish. When wrapped, these foods can be a fun, creative, fresh, and healthful meal. And they make a great meal on the go. Once you know how to create your own wraps, you can do a meal for a car trip or an outdoor summer concert. Wraps also make great appetizers. They are quick and simple, and you can make the filling days ahead. Your guests will have something to eat when they arrive. Many of the dishes can be served as appetizers or main dishes. You will find that a number of the recipes in this chapter combine Asian and western ingredients and cooking techniques.

New Year's Dumpling Delight

You can be creative and adventurous with dumplings. Feel free to substitute some of your own favorite ingredients in the filling and sauce. You may want to use hot chili oil instead of sesame oil to add zing to the sauce. For the filling, you can experiment with seasoned mashed potatoes, tofu, lean pork, or smoked salmon. Or make some wild creation such as a sweet fruit filling and serve the dumplings as a novel dessert. You can make the filling ahead of time. It will keep in the refrigerator for 2 days or in the freezer for up to 1 week.

Traditionally, the steamer basket (pages 44–45) is heavily coated with oil to keep the dumplings from sticking. I've found a delightful alternative. Take a plump, round carrot and thinly slice it into disks. Place each dumpling on its own disk. When the dumplings come out of the steamer, each has its own little serving tray. As a bonus, the carrot becomes sweet and tender during steaming. My son loves to eat his dumpling trays.

FILLING

¾ POUND LEAN GROUND PORK OR BEEF

1 TABLESPOON LOW-SODIUM SOY SAUCE

1 TABLESPOON CANOLA OIL

4 LARGE NAPA CABBAGE LEAVES, ABOUT 5 OUNCES

2 GREEN ONIONS (GREEN AND WHITE PARTS), MINCED

4 FRESH SHIITAKE MUSHROOMS, MINCED

1 TABLESPOON MINCED FRESH GINGER

1 CUP MINCED LEEKS (WHITE PART ONLY)

1 TABLESPOON RICE WINE

¼ TEASPOON PEPPER

DASH OF SALT

2 TEASPOONS SESAME OIL

2 LARGE, THICK CARROTS

40 SQUARE WONTON WRAPPERS (SEE PAGE 63)

1 CUP GINGER AND GARLIC SAUCE (PAGE 79)

Make the filling: In a large bowl, mix the meat, soy sauce, and oil. Set aside.

Trim stems off cabbage leaves and discard. Mince the leaves. Squeeze out the liquid from the minced cabbage. Mix it in with the meat filling.

Combine the remaining filling ingredients with the meat mixture in the large bowl. Mix well.

Thinly slice the carrots into disks. You'll need one disk for each wonton.

Set up a space for folding the dumplings. Place a bowl of cold water, the wonton wrappers, the filling, and the steamer basket around your workspace. Cover wrappers with a moist paper towel to prevent drying. Place the carrot slices in the steamer.

With each wrapper, dip all four edges into the cold water. Holding the wrapper flat on your palm, place about one teaspoon of filling in the center of the wrapper. Bring the four corners of the wrapper up over the filling. Pinch the edges together tightly. Set each dumpling on a carrot slice, leaving a little space between each dumpling.

Add enough water to a pot for steaming but not enough to touch the steamer basket. Bring the water to a boil. Set the steamer over the water. Steam until dumpling skins are translucent, 10 to 12 minutes.

Serve with the sauce for dipping.

Makes 40 dumplings

TIPS

THERE SHOULD BE ADEQUATE WATER IN THE POT TO BOIL FOR SEVERAL MINUTES, BUT IT SHOULD NOT TOUCH THE DUMPLINGS IN THE STEAMER.

IF YOU DON'T HAVE A STEAMER BASKET, YOU CAN USE A HEATPROOF PLATE. ELEVATE THE PLATE WITH A HEATPROOF BOWL ON THE BOTTOM OF THE POT. ADD WATER TO THE POT. FILL THE BOWL WITH WATER AND PLACE THE PLATE ON TOP. COVER AND STEAM.

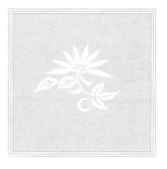

Green Tea–Steamed Tofu-Mushroom Dumplings

Most of the dumplings served at Chinese restaurants are made with meat. In China, one of the most popular dumpling fillings is made with tofu and mushrooms.

FILLING

1 POUND FIRM TOFU

1 TABLESPOON CANOLA OIL

1 TABLESPOON MINCED FRESH GINGER

1 CUP MINCED FRESH OR DRIED MUSHROOMS CAPS

1 TABLESPOON RICE WINE

2½ TABLESPOONS SOY SAUCE

1½ TABLESPOONS SESAME OIL

1 TEASPOON GROUND WHITE PEPPER

40 SQUARE WONTON WRAPPERS (SEE PAGE 63)

2 PLUMP CARROTS, CUT INTO 40 THIN DISKS

6 BAGS GREEN TEA

SPICY LEMON-BASIL SAUCE (PAGE 83)

Make the filling: Place the tofu on a cutting board or flat surface and press out the excess water. Use a large spoon or your hand to break tofu into fine crumbs.

Heat the oil in a small skillet over medium heat. Add the ginger and sauté until lightly browned, about 1 minute. Add the mushrooms and sauté until soft, about 2 minutes.

Combine the mushrooms and tofu and the remaining filling ingredients in a large bowl. Mix thoroughly.

Set up a space for folding the dumplings. Place a bowl of cold water, the wonton wrappers, the filling, and a steamer basket around your workspace. Cover wrappers with a damp paper towel to prevent drying. Arrange the carrot rounds in the steamer.

With each wrapper, dip all four edges into the cold water. Holding the wrapper flat on your palm, place about 1 heaping teaspoon of the filling in the center. Bring the four corners of the wrapper up over the filling. Pinch the edges together tightly. Set each dumpling on a carrot round, leaving a little space between them.

In a large pot, bring 5 to 6 cups water to a boil. Add the tea bags. Place the dumplings over the boiling tea. Make sure the water doesn't reach the dumplings (see Tips, page 107). Cover and steam over high heat until dumpling skins are translucent, 10 to 12 minutes. Serve warm with sauce.

Makes 40 dumplings

Pan-Fried Shrimp Dumplings

Pan-fried, crisp, dumplings don't have to be loaded with fat. By using water and oil together, I've found that they come out not only crisp on the bottom, but also soft and juicy on top and inside.

FILLING

¾ POUND MEDIUM RAW SHRIMP, PEELED, DEVEINED, AND MINCED

4 GREEN ONIONS (WHITE PART ONLY), MINCED

4 CLOVES GARLIC, MINCED

1½ TABLESPOONS MINCED FRESH GINGER

2 TABLESPOONS SOY SAUCE

1 TABLESPOON RICE WINE OR WHITE WINE

1 TEASPOON CHILI PEPPER OIL

40 ROUND (GYOZA) DUMPLING WRAPPERS (PAGE 53)

2 TABLESPOONS CANOLA OIL

½ CUP WATER

½ CUP ORANGE AND SOY SAUCE (PAGE 89)

Make the filling: In a bowl, combine all the filling ingredients and mix well.

Set up a space for folding the dumplings. Place a bowl of cold water, the wrappers, and the filling around your workspace. Cover the wrappers, with a damp towel to prevent drying. Dip one edge of a wrapper into the water. Place 1 heaping teaspoon of filling in the center of the wrapper. Fold the wrapper over to form a half-circle, joining the dry edge to the wet edge. Pinch the edges together to seal the dumpling.

Put 1 tablespoon of the oil and ¼ cup of the water in a large non-stick skillet. Place half of the dumplings in a spiraling circle in the pan, leaving just a little space between each one. Cover and cook over medium heat until dumplings puff up and are a light brown on the bottom, 8 to 10 minutes. Repeat with the remaining dumplings, oil, and water.

Serve the warm dumplings with the Orange and Soy Sauce.

Makes 40 dumplings

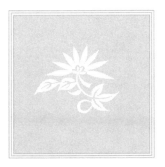

Spicy Shrimp and Vegetables in Lettuce Cups

This is a delightful dish. The crisp, colorful vegetables complement the spicy shrimp beautifully. You can also substitute tofu or lean meat for the shrimp.

MARINADE

1 SMALL FRESH RED CAYENNE PEPPER, MINCED

3 CLOVES GARLIC, MINCED

2 TEASPOONS MINCED FRESH GINGER

1 TABLESPOON COOKING WINE

2 TABLESPOONS FISH SAUCE (PAGE 53)

¾ POUND BABY SHRIMP

2 HEADS ICEBERG LETTUCE

3 TABLESPOONS SAVORY OIL (PAGE 81)

½ CUP RED ONION, DICED SMALL

½ CUP LEEK (WHITE PART ONLY), MINCED

½ CUP DICED CARROT

1 TABLESPOON RICE VINEGAR (PAGE 57)

1½ TABLESPOONS LOW-SODIUM SOY SAUCE

1 CUP DICED RED BELL PEPPER

SALT AND PEPPER TO TASTE

½ CUP PINE NUTS, TOASTED (SEE TIPS, PAGE 96)

1 TEASPOON SESAME OIL

2 GREEN ONIONS (GREEN AND WHITE PARTS), MINCED

LETTUCE (ROMAINE, BOSTON, ICEBERG, OR ANY LEAFY LETTUCE)

I HAVE FOUND THAT USING LETTUCE LEAVES AS WRAPPERS IS A GREAT WAY TO ADD EXTRA VEGETABLES TO YOUR DIET AND CUT DOWN ON CARBOHYDRATES. THEIR CRISP TEXTURE GOES WELL WITH ANY FILLING. LEAFY, GREEN LETTUCES ARE IDEAL FOR ROLL-UP DISHES. BOSTON AND ICEBERG LETTUCES CREATE PERFECT "CUPS." IF YOUR CHILDREN ENJOY WRAPPING THEIR OWN FOOD, THIS IS A GREAT WAY TO SNEAK SOME LETTUCE INTO THEIR MEAL.

Mix all the marinade ingredients in a small bowl. Add the shrimp and marinate for 2 hours in the refrigerator.

Cut out the lettuce cores and separate the leaves. Cut the leaves into 4-inch squares to make "cups." Arrange the lettuce on a large serving plate.

Coat a nonstick cooking pan with the oil, and heat over medium-high heat. Add the onion and leek and stir-fry until fragrant, about 30 seconds. Add the carrot and stir-fry for 1 minute. Add the rice vinegar, soy sauce, and red bell pepper. Stir-fry for 30 seconds. Mix in the shrimp, including the marinade. Stir-fry until shrimp are heated through, about 1 minute. Season with salt and pepper. Remove from heat.

Toss in the pine nuts, sesame oil, and green onions. To serve, spoon 2 tablespoons of the mixture into a lettuce leaf cup, wrap, and eat by hand.

Makes about 24 lettuce cups

Meatballs in Spicy Ginger-Coconut Sauce

These meatballs are perfect for any occasion. Make them ahead of time, and keep them chilled or frozen until you are ready to cook them.

SAUCE

1 CUP REDUCED-FAT, UNSWEETENED COCONUT MILK (SEE PAGE 52)

5 QUARTER-SIZE GINGER SLICES

2 TABLESPOONS FISH SAUCE (SEE PAGE 53)

1 TABLESPOON HONEY

MEATBALLS

1 POUND LEAN GROUND PORK OR GROUND BEEF

1 EGG, LIGHTLY BEATEN

1 TABLESPOON SESAME OIL

1 TABLESPOON MINCED GINGER

2 GREEN ONIONS (GREEN AND WHITE PARTS), CHOPPED

5 SPRIGS CILANTRO, MINCED

1 FRESH RED CAYENNE PEPPER, FINELY CHOPPED

¼ TEASPOON SALT

1 TEASPOON WHITE PEPPER

2 TABLESPOONS CANOLA OIL

FISH SAUCE (OPTIONAL)

FRESH RED CHILI PEPPER, MINCED (OPTIONAL)

¼ CUP BASIL LEAVES, CHOPPED

1 TABLESPOON GRATED LEMON PEEL

7 (8-INCH) FLOUR TORTILLAS, WARMED (PAGE 115)

TORTILLAS

TORTILLAS ARE MADE WITH FLOUR OR CORN AND AVAILABLE IN 6-, 8- AND 10-INCH SIZES. THE IMPORTANT THING TO REMEMBER IS TO ALWAYS HEAT THE TORTILLAS SO THEY WILL BE SOFT AND PLIABLE TO WRAP AROUND THE FILLING WITHOUT CRACKING. YOU CAN BUY THEM AT MOST GROCERY STORES. LOOK FOR TORTILLAS THAT ARE LOW IN SODIUM.

THREE EASY WAYS TO HEAT TORTILLAS

MICROWAVE: STACK THE TORTILLAS BETWEEN TWO DAMP PAPER TOWELS AND MICROWAVE FOR 8 TO 10 SECONDS, UNTIL HOT AND PLIABLE.

OVEN: PREHEAT THE OVEN TO 300°F (150°C) WHILE YOU PREPARE THE FILLING. STACK THE TORTILLAS, FOUR AT A TIME, BETWEEN TWO DAMP PAPER TOWELS. WRAP TIGHTLY WITH FOIL. PLACE THEM IN THE OVEN FOR 4 TO 6 MINUTES, OR UNTIL WARM.

STEAM: SPRAY TORTILLAS WITH CANOLA OIL AND FOLD INTO QUARTERS. PLACE THEM IN A DEEP PLATE. STEAM ON A RACK OVER BOILING WATER FOR 5 MINUTES.

Make the sauce: Mix all the ingredients in a bowl and set aside.

Make the meatballs: Place all the ingredients in a large bowl. Knead well by hand until the ingredients are thoroughly combined and the mixture becomes sticky. Divide the mixture into 14 equal portions, about 2 tablespoons each. Roll each portion into a ball. Set meatballs on an oiled plate.

Heat the canola oil in a nonstick cooking pan over medium-high heat, swirling to coat the sides. Add the meatballs, and fry, turning occasionally, until browned on all sides, 7 to 10 minutes.

Add the sauce. Cover and simmer for 8 to 10 minutes. Taste, and adjust the seasonings with fish sauce and chili pepper, if using.

Sprinkle with basil leaves and lemon peel. Wrap two meatballs and sauce in each flour tortilla. Serve hot.

Makes 7 servings

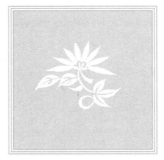

Seared Steak with Cucumber and Mango

The first time I was served pork chops and applesauce, I didn't like it. But I couldn't help experimenting with my own meat and fruit combinations. This mild cucumber/hot-flavored steak/sweet mango wrap is unforgettable.

1 POUND BEEF FLANK STEAK

MARINADE

¼ CUP FRESH ORANGE JUICE

2 TABLESPOONS EXTRA-VIRGIN OLIVE OIL

1 TEASPOON FRESHLY GROUND BLACK PEPPER

¼ TEASPOON GARLIC SALT

¼ CUP CILANTRO LEAVES, MINCED

6 (10-INCH) FLOUR TORTILLAS, WARMED (SEE PAGE 115)

2 MEDIUM MANGOES, PEELED, SEEDED, AND CUT INTO STRIPS

1 ENGLISH CUCUMBER, PEELED AND CUT INTO STRIPS

Using a sharp knife, trim any fat or gristle off the steak. Cut the steak into 1-inch slices.

Make the marinade: Mix all the ingredients in a bowl. Add the steak and marinate overnight in the refrigerator.

Preheat the oven to broil, and broil the steak on a broiler pan until desired doneness. Let stand for 5 minutes. Cut meat across the grain into thin strips.

Lay the warmed tortillas on a work surface, and arrange some of the meat, mangoes, and cucumber on top. Roll up, and enjoy.

Makes 4 to 6 servings

Spicy Coconut Meatballs in Pita Bread

Make the meatballs ahead of time and keep them chilled or frozen until you are ready to cook them. They will keep in the refrigerator for up to 5 days. Throughout the week, simply mix and match them with your favorite vegetables or fruit.

SAUCE

½ CUP SOYMILK

½ CUP REDUCED-FAT, UNSWEETENED COCONUT MILK (SEE PAGE 52)

1 TABLESPOON COCONUT-FLAVORED YOGURT

2 TEASPOONS FISH SAUCE (SEE PAGE 53)

5 SPRIGS CILANTRO, CHOPPED

1 RED CHILI, CHOPPED

1 TABLESPOON GRATED LEMON PEEL

MEATBALLS

½ CUP WATER

2 TEASPOONS LOOSE GREEN TEA

½ POUND LEAN GROUND PORK OR GROUND BEEF

2 TABLESPOONS SOY SAUCE

½ TABLESPOON GRATED LEMON PEEL

1 TEASPOON SESAME OIL

1 TABLESPOON MINCED GINGER

5 SPRIGS CILANTRO, MINCED

1 FRESH GREEN OR RED CHILI, FINELY CHOPPED

1 TABLESPOON CORNSTARCH

1 TABLESPOON ALL-PURPOSE FLOUR

1 TABLESPOON CANOLA OIL

4 PITA BREADS

½ CUP RED BELL PEPPER STRIPS, GRILLED

½ CUP SNOW PEAS, GRILLED

PITA BREAD

THIS IS A ROUND, LEAVENED WHEAT FLOUR BREAD FROM THE MIDDLE EAST. IT FORMS A NATURAL POCKET WHILE BAKING. IT COMES IN DIFFERENT SIZES. YOU CAN FIND IT AT WELL-STOCKED GROCERY STORES AND SPECIALTY FOOD MARKETS. IT'S VERY FILLING AND GOES WELL WITH MEATS AND VEGETABLES.

Make the sauce: Mix all the sauce ingredients in a bowl and set aside.

Make the meatballs: Bring the water to a boil. Pour over the tea. Let it brew for 3 minutes. Reserve the tea leaves (drink the tea after you add some more hot water). Mince the tea leaves.

In a large bowl, mix the meat and soy sauce thoroughly. Add the tea and remaining meatball ingredients and mix well. Divide mixture into 16 equal portions, about 2 tablespoons each. Roll each portion into a ball.

Heat a wide nonstick frying pan over medium-high heat. Add the oil, swirling to coat sides. Add the meatballs and fry, turning occasionally, until browned on all sides, 7 to 10 minutes. Add the sauce. Cover and simmer for 8 to 10 minutes.

To serve, cut open one end of each pita loaf and open the pockets. Spoon 4 meatballs and some grilled vegetables into each pita pocket and eat with your fingers.

Makes 4 servings

Lion's Head

This is a well-known Chinese dish made with ground meat and napa cabbage. The reheated rolls taste even better after having a chance to soak up all the sauce. The recipe can be doubled.

1 LARGE HEAD NAPA CABBAGE, OUTER LEAVES DISCARDED

6 CUPS WATER

2 GREEN TEA BAGS

¾ POUND LEAN GROUND PORK

2 TABLESPOONS SOY SAUCE

¼ CUP GREEN ONIONS (GREEN AND WHITE PARTS), FINELY MINCED

1 TABLESPOON FINELY MINCED GINGER

¼ CUP FINELY MINCED FRESH OR DRIED SHIITAKE MUSHROOM CAPS

1 TABLESPOON RICE WINE

1 TABLESPOON SESAME OIL

1 TABLESPOON CORNSTARCH

1 TABLESPOON ALL-PURPOSE FLOUR

4 CUPS VEGETABLE AND MUSHROOM STOCK (PAGE 73), GINSENG-CHICKEN STOCK (PAGE 69), OR CANNED STOCK

SALT AND WHITE PEPPER TO TASTE

COOKED RICE OR NOODLES

Separate the cabbage into individual leaves. Wash and drain. In a large pot, bring 4 cups water to a boil. Add the tea bags. Add the leaves and boil until leaves soften, about 1 minute. Remove the leaves with a strainer and rinse under cold water. Drain the leaves and cut the stem sections from the leaves into 3- to 4-inch squares.

In a large bowl, mix the meat and soy sauce thoroughly with a large spoon or by hand. Add the onions, ginger, mushrooms, rice wine, sesame oil, cornstarch, and flour. Mix until smooth and sticky.

Place about 2 tablespoons meat mixture into the center of a cabbage leaf. Fold the left and right side over the filling. Then, starting at the bottom, roll the leaves up to form a neatly filled pocket. Repeat with the remaining filling and cabbage leaves.

In a large casserole or pot, place the cabbage rolls folded side down. Add the stock and bring to a boil. Add the cabbage stems, and bring to a second boil. Turn down heat to medium-low and partially cover the pot. Simmer until half of the stock cooks off, about 40 minutes. Season with salt and pepper. Serve cabbage rolls with the broth over rice or noodles.

Makes 6 servings

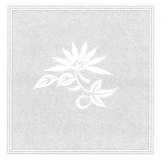

Fresh Spring Rolls

I have found that no other appetizers at a party get as much attention as this one. It is also a good lunch for summer outings. Feel free to replace the tofu with shrimp or chicken.

FILLING

2 TABLESPOONS SAVORY OIL (PAGE 81)

½ TABLESPOONS MINCED GARLIC

8 OUNCES FLAVORED, BAKED TOFU (PACKAGED,
    OR FOLLOW THE RECIPE ON PAGE 125), SHREDDED

1 CUP SHREDDED FRESH MUSHROOMS CAPS

4 GREEN ONIONS (GREEN PART ONLY), CUT INTO
    SHORT THIN SLIVERS

1 MEDIUM RED BELL PEPPER, CUT INTO SHORT
    THIN STRIPS

½ TABLESPOON SESAME OIL

1 TABLESPOON RICE VINEGAR (PAGE 58)

SALT AND WHITE PEPPER TO TASTE

12 (8-INCH) ROUND DRIED RICE PAPER WRAPPERS

1 CUP GREEN CHILI SAUCE (PAGE 92)
    OR THAI SAUCE (PAGE 91)

Make the filling: Heat a nonstick frying pan over medium-high heat. Add the oil, swirling to coat sides. Add the garlic and sauté until fragrant, about 30 seconds. Add the tofu, mushrooms, green onions, and red pepper. Stir-fry for 1 minute. Stir in the sesame oil and vinegar. Season with salt and pepper.

Soak a sheet of rice paper wrapper in warm water until soft, about 1 minute. Carefully transfer the wrapper to a dry cutting board.

Arrange 2 tablespoons of the filling in an even horizontal mound just below the center of the wrapper. Tightly roll up the rice paper to form a tight cylinder, folding in the sides about halfway, as you would to form an egg roll or a blintz. Assemble the remaining spring rolls the same way. Cut each spring roll in half on the diagonal.

Serve with the sauce for dipping.

Makes 12 rolls

RICE WRAPPERS

THESE ARE ROUND OR TRIANGULAR TRANSLUCENT SHEETS MADE FROM RICE FLOUR. THEY ARE WIDELY USED IN VIETNAMESE AND THAI COOKING. ONCE DIPPED IN HOT WATER, THE DELICATE, DRY SHEETS BECOME SOFT AND PLIABLE IN SECONDS. WHEN YOU HAVE WORKED WITH THEM A FEW TIMES, THEY BECOME VERY EASY TO MASTER. ONCE OPENED, STORE THEM IN AIRTIGHT PLASTIC BAGS. IF STORED IN A COOL, DRY PLACE, THEY WILL KEEP ABOUT 2 MONTHS. RICE WRAPPERS GO WELL WITH FRESH VEGETABLES AND SEAFOOD, ALONG WITH A DIPPING SAUCE.

Tofu Hand-Roll

This dish was inspired by one eaten at a Japanese restaurant in China. You may replace the tofu with grilled fish or shrimp, or substitute small pita pockets for nori.

¼ CUP CANOLA OIL

1 TABLESPOON LOOSE GREEN TEA, PREFERABLY GUNPOWDER

1 CUP FINELY CHOPPED OYSTER MUSHROOMS

8 OUNCES FLAVORED, BAKED TOFU, FINELY CHOPPED INTO CUBES

½ CUP FINELY CUBED CARROT

½ CUP FINELY CUBED GREEN APPLE

½ CUP FINELY CHOPPED CANNED WATER CHESTNUTS

1 CUP SPICY LEMON-BASIL SAUCE (PAGE 83)

SALT AND PEPPER TO TASTE

1½ TABLESPOONS MINCED PICKLED GINGER

2 GREEN ONIONS (GREEN AND WHITE PARTS), MINCED

2 TEASPOONS SESAME OIL

12 (10 X 7 X 8-INCH) SHEETS TOASTED NORI

SPICY SESAME SAUCE (PAGE 78), TO SERVE

Heat a nonstick wok or skillet over medium heat. Add the canola oil and swirl to coat. Add the tea and stir-fry until fragrant, about 30 seconds. Add the mushrooms and tofu and stir-fry for 2 minutes. Add carrot, apple, and water chestnuts and stir-fry for 30 seconds.

Add the Spicy Lemon-Basil Sauce. Cook, stirring occasionally, until vegetables are heated through, about 2 minutes. Season with salt and pepper. Remove from heat. Add the pickled ginger, green onions, and sesame oil, and toss to combine.

To serve, roll a nori sheet into a cone, glossy side out. Spoon 4 tablespoons of the mixture into the cone and eat out of your hand. Serve with the Spicy Sesame Sauce for dipping.

Makes 12 appetizers

Teriyaki Tofu

To make your own baked seasoned tofu, try the following recipe:

CONTENTS OF 2 GINSENG OR GREEN TEA BAGS

1 (16-OUNCE) BLOCK EXTRA-FIRM OR LOW-FAT FRESH TOFU

1 CUP TERIYAKI SAUCE (PAGE 90) OR PURCHASED

1 ½ TABLESPOONS FRESH LEMON JUICE

1 TABLESPOON MINCED GINGER

Combine the tea (discard the tea bags), Teriyaki Sauce, lemon juice, and ginger in a plastic container. Place a small plate on top of the tofu and gently press out the water. Slice the tofu lengthwise in half. Marinate in the sauce overnight, making sure the sauce covers the tofu. Bake the tofu on a baking sheet at 350°F (175°C) for 30 minutes, or until the tofu is firm and compact.

Mu Shu Tofu

This is one of the most famous Chinese dishes in the United States. Almost every Chinese restaurant I visit has a mu shu dish on the menu. Most of time it's mu shu chicken. But there is no reason that vegetarian lovers can't enjoy mu shu, too. I created this version to show just how versatile this dish can be. It makes a great lunch.

2 EGGS

1 GREEN ONION (GREEN AND WHITE PARTS), MINCED

1 TABLESPOON MINCED FRESH GINGER

1 TABLESPOON SAVORY OIL (PAGE 81) OR PURCHASED

¼ TEASPOON SALT

½ TEASPOON WHITE PEPPER

3 TABLESPOONS CANOLA OIL

2 CLOVES GARLIC, CHOPPED

8 OUNCES FLAVORED, BAKED TOFU (PACKAGED, OR RECIPE ON PAGE 125),
    THINLY SHREDDED

1 CUP FRESH OR DRIED SHIITAKE MUSHROOM CAPS, THINLY SHREDDED

½ CUP LEEK (WHITE PART ONLY), THINLY SHREDDED

1 TABLESPOON RICE WINE

SALT AND PEPPER TO TASTE

4 (8-INCH) FLOUR TORTILLAS, WARMED (SEE PAGE 115)

½ CUP ROASTED RED PEPPER–SUN-DRIED TOMATOES SAUCE (PAGE 100)

In a bowl, lightly beat the eggs, mix in the green onion, ginger, Savory Oil, salt, and pepper. Beat the egg mixture until light and fluffy.

Heat a nonstick skillet over medium heat. Add 2 tablespoons of the canola oil and swirl to coat. Pour in egg mixture. Don't scramble. Let it set and brown on the bottom, turn, and brown the other side. Remove from heat and cut into long strips.

Heat the remaining oil in the skillet, add the garlic, and sauté until fragrant. Add the tofu, mushrooms, and leek and stir-fry for 2 minutes. Add the rice wine and season with salt and pepper.

To serve, place the tortillas on a serving plate, spread 2 tablespoons of Roasted Red Pepper–Sun-Dried Tomatoes Sauce over each tortilla, spoon some of the tofu mixture on top, and top with egg strips. Roll up and eat with your fingers.

Makes 4 servings

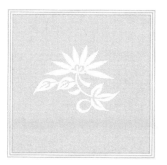

Crabmeat-Spinach Ravioli

Although you can buy ravioli with all kinds of fillings, a few times I have found that the filling is too salty and heavy. I always have fun making them at home.

1 POUND FRESH SPINACH LEAVES

½ CUP FRESH OR FROZEN CRABMEAT, PICKED OVER

4 CLOVES GARLIC, FINELY MINCED

1 CUP RICOTTA CHEESE

SALT AND PEPPER TO TASTE

FRESH PASTA SHEETS

1½ CUPS ROASTED PEPPER–SUN-DRIED TOMATOES
    SAUCE (PAGE 100), HEATED

In a large pot, bring 4 cups water to a boil. Add the spinach and boil until wilted. Rinse under cold water. Use your hand to squeeze out the water.

In a large bowl, combine the spinach, crabmeat, garlic, and cheese, and season with salt and pepper.

Cut pasta sheets into long strips about 4 inches wide. Place 2 teaspoons of filling down the center for the length of the strips, leaving about 2 inches between dollops. Brush water around the edges. Cover with another strip. Press down the top strip and press out any air inside the pockets. Cut between the rows with a small sharp knife to form small squares with the filling in the center of each.

Place the ravioli on a floured work surface. Let them air-dry on both sides.

In a big pot, bring 5 cups water to a boil. Drop ravioli, one at a time, in boiling water. Simmer until raviolis start floating to the top.

Drain and arrange them in serving plates. Spoon the sauce on top. Serve hot.

Makes 4 servings

CHINESE DINING CUSTOMS

+ LET THE HOST OR HOSTESS LEAD THE WAY TO THE TABLE.
+ SIT AT THE APPOINTED SEAT.
+ DON'T START TO EAT UNTIL THE HOST OR HOSTESS STARTS AND INVITES EVERYBODY TO JOIN. THIS ALSO APPLIES TO EVERY NEW DISH BROUGHT TO THE TABLE.
+ BE PREPARED TO MAKE AT LEAST THREE TOASTS.
+ OFFER TO FILL GLASSES AND TEACUPS FOR PERSONS SITTING NEXT TO YOU.
+ THE MEAL ENDS WHEN THE HOST OR HOSTESS AND THE GUEST OF HONOR RISE.

Avocado Bruschetta with Roasted Pepper Sauce

You can prepare the roasted pepper sauce ahead of time, but make the avocado mixture and toast the bread just before serving for the best color and taste. If you have trouble finding orange and yellow tomatoes, substitute cherry tomatoes.

1 LARGE RIPE HAAS AVOCADO, PITTED, PEELED,
 AND CUT INTO ½-INCH CHUNKS

1 SMALL ORANGE TOMATO, CUT INTO ½-INCH CHUNKS

2 SMALL YELLOW TOMATOES, CUT INTO ½-INCH CHUNKS

1 TABLESPOON FRESH LEMON JUICE

1 TABLESPOON EXTRA-VIRGIN OLIVE OIL

SALT TO TASTE

1½ CUPS ROASTED PEPPER–SUN-DRIED TOMATOES
 SAUCE (PAGE 100) OR PESTO SAUCE (PAGE 96)

20 (½-INCH-THICK) SLICES SOURDOUGH FLUTE
 (LONG, SKINNY BREAD, FOUND IN MOST GROCERY
 STORES), LIGHTLY TOASTED

In a medium bowl, toss the avocado, tomato chunks, lemon juice, and olive oil. Season with salt.

Using a knife, spread about 1 tablespoon of the sauce on each slice of bread. Arrange the avocado mixture on top. Serve immediately.

Makes 20 servings

Broiled Shiitake Mushroom Sandwiches

The longer you marinate the mushrooms, the better the flavor. If you can, marinate them overnight.

1 POUND MEDIUM FRESH SHIITAKE MUSHROOMS OR 20 DRIED

1½ CUPS APPLE-ORANGE SAUCE (PAGE 98) OR TERIYAKI SAUCE (PAGE 90)

1 LARGE ENGLISH CUCUMBER, THINLY SLICED

2 MEDIUM TOMATOES, THINLY SLICED

For fresh mushrooms, wash and discard the stems. For dried mushrooms, soak the mushrooms in warm water until softened, about 15 minutes; drain. Discard stems.

Combine all the marinade ingredients in a bowl. Mix well. Spoon on top of the mushroom caps. Cover and refrigerate for 30 minutes or longer.

Preheat the broiler. Place mushroom caps, stem sides up, in a greased baking pan. Spray lightly with cooking spray.

Broil with the tops 4 inches from heat until light brown, 5 to 6 minutes.

Arrange cucumber slices on a plate. Place a mushroom on each cucumber slice, then top with a tomato slice.

Makes 20 sandwiches

Pan-Fried Tofu with Mango-Ginger Salsa

This is a great dish for introducing tofu to those meat lovers in your life.

2 (6-OUNCE) PACKAGES FLAVORED, BAKED TOFU

3 TABLESPOONS CANOLA OIL

2 CLOVES GARLIC, MINCED

1½ CUPS MANGO-GINGER SALSA (PAGE 99)

Put the tofu on a flat surface, place a plate on top, and gently press the water from the tofu.

Cut each tofu block horizontally to make 2 sheets. Slice each sheet, making a total of 12 thin rectangular pieces.

Heat 1½ tablespoons of the oil in a nonstick cooking pan over medium-high heat and swirl to coat pan. Add the garlic and sauté until fragrant, about 30 seconds. Line the bottom of the pan with the tofu sheets. Pan-fry until golden brown. Add the remaining 1½ tablespoons oil, turn, and pan-fry the other side, about 3 minutes on each side.

Place tofu on a serving plate. Top with Mango-Ginger Salsa. Eat with your fingers.

Makes 8 servings

5. Meals in a Pot: Soups, Stews, and Hot Pots

For me, the pleasures of soup have always been associated with feelings of warmth, relaxation, and comfort. Soups and stews are healthy, nurturing, easy, and delicious. The Chinese consider soups to be a vital way of receiving the health benefits of one's food. The slow process of cooking the soup stock or soup gives the ingredients a chance to release all the flavors and mingle together for the most delicious taste.

The keys to success of soup and stew are in the stock and a good combination of fresh ingredients. Use homemade stock (pages 69 to 77) or organic canned stock as a base for the soup. You can also make many of the recipes ahead of time and freeze them. They can be heated for a delicious meal on a busy weeknight. Use fresh, organic meat for the stew.

Most of these dishes call for healthy Asian ingredients, but in small amounts. By making these ingredients a regular part of your diet, the cumulative effect of small amounts provides all the long-term health benefits you need. The longer cooking time of soups and stews releases more of the benefits of the healthy ingredients into the dish.

Soups are also a great solution to take care of leftovers. In a way, your leftovers have already been "stewing" in the refrigerator as their flavors mingle. Remember to include them in your next stew or soup.

In this chapter you will find thick broths and stews, which can be meals in themselves; light soup can be served as starter, or make a full meal by adding a salad, rice, or bread.

Lemongrass-Coconut-Flavored Tofu Soup is a warming appetizer. Try a relaxing bowl of Hot and Sour Shrimp Soup on a hot summer day. Whether you feel sick or just run-down, Chicken-Ginseng Soup is the ideal comfort food.

In my hometown of Wuhan in central China, winter becomes an endless parade of days that are chilly, gray, and damp. Yet I always looked forward to mealtime, because Grandmother made hot soup for us.

Hot Pots

On weekends Grandmother always made a hot pot. This was one of my favorites. I watched Grandmother slice meat, boil fish balls, and cut tofu. Her skillful knife turned bamboo shoots into miniature trees, green onions into bushes, tomatoes into roses, and carrots and icicle radishes into flowers.

Making a hot pot involved the entire family. As Grandmother prepared the ingredients, I helped arrange them on serving plates. My brothers helped my father light the charcoal stove. Mother put broth in a sand pot and prepared the dipping sauces for everyone.

Sitting before the fire on long winter nights and sharing a hot pot with my family were some of the happiest moments of my childhood.

Hot pot aficionados traditionally use a sand pot, a ceramic pot with a rough, unglazed exterior and a glazed interior. First, broth is boiled in the pot over a small charcoal stove in the center of the table.

You may find it more practical to use a casserole dish set over a gas or alcohol burner or an electric hot plate. If you don't have any of these, I've found that an electric wok or fondue set will work just as well. You can bring the broth to a boil in a large pot in the kitchen and carefully pour it into the pot for cooking.

Hot pot cooking time is very short. You will need to prepare all the ingredients in advance. Arrange them artistically on the serving plates.

Once the broth in the hot pot is boiling, everyone cooks his or her own ingredients. Try not to overcook. Vegetables only need to be scalded so they are heated through. Tofu, mushrooms, and meat need a little longer, about 1 minute. Be sure to use the dipping sauce before eating. Diners flavor the broth as they cook their meal. Toward the end, divide up and enjoy the well-seasoned broth. Each person should have a large slotted spoon or chopsticks to move the food to and from the hot pot, and small, shallow bowls for dipping sauces. Each diner is provided with a plate.

If you are pressed for time, you can cook all the ingredients together, and serve hot pot soup; see Tofu Hot Pot (page 137).

Chicken-Ginseng Soup

In China, soup is not served as a course. It's intended to be a beverage consumed with the meal. The Chinese believe that cold drinks are harmful to your digestive system. This flavorful, light soup will accompany your other dishes well. The ginseng in the soup is considered to have calming and cleansing effects.

2 TABLESPOONS CANOLA OIL

2 TABLESPOONS ¼-INCH FRESH GINGER CHUNKS

6 CLOVES GARLIC, MINCED

1 MEDIUM ONION, CUBED

1 POUND BONELESS, SKINLESS CHICKEN BREASTS,
    CUT INTO 1-INCH CHUNKS

3 CUPS SPRING WATER

6 CUPS CANNED LOW-SODIUM, LOW-FAT CHICKEN BROTH

2 WHOLE OR SLICED AMERICAN GINSENG ROOTS
    (ABOUT ½ OUNCE) OR 4 GINSENG TEA BAGS

3 CUPS FRESH OR FROZEN WHOLE-KERNEL CORN

SALT AND WHITE PEPPER TO TASTE

Heat a nonstick wok or skillet over medium heat and coat it with the oil. Add the ginger, garlic, and onion and sauté until fragrant, 1 to 2 minutes. Add the chicken and sauté until the chicken browns slightly, 2 to 3 minutes.

In a big pot, bring the water and chicken broth to a boil. Add the chicken mixture, ginseng, and corn. Bring to a second boil. Reduce the heat and simmer for 20 minutes. Season with salt and pepper. Remove ginseng tea bags, if using. If using ginseng root, eat as desired.

Makes 5½ cups

Tofu Hot Pot

This has been my favorite vegetarian soup since childhood. It's so delicious and filling, it's a meal in itself. Freezing and thawing the tofu helps keep it firm and gives it a pleasant, chewier texture. It also makes the tofu more porous, so it soaks up the flavors of the soup better. But you don't have to freeze the tofu if you don't have time.

1 (16-OUNCE) PACKAGE EXTRA-FIRM TOFU

½ POUND DRIED RICE NOODLES OR BEAN THREAD NOODLES (PAGE 55)

5 CUPS BOILING WATER

1 CUP TERIYAKI SAUCE (PAGE 90) OR PURCHASED

1 CUP SNOW PEAS

½ POUND BABY BOK CHOY (CHINESE CABBAGE) OR NAPA CABBAGE,
    CUT INTO 4-INCH SQUARES

1 RED BELL PEPPER, CUT INTO 2-INCH SQUARES

1 YELLOW BELL PEPPER, CUT INTO 2-INCH SQUARES

BROTH

6 CUPS VEGETABLE AND MUSHROOM STOCK (PAGE 73), SPICY VEGETABLE
    STOCK (PAGE 71) OR CANNED VEGETABLE STOCK

2 CUPS SPRING WATER

½ GINSENG ROOT OR 4 GINSENG SLICES

2 TABLESPOONS COOKING WINE

2 TEASPOONS SALT

4 TABLESPOONS LOW-SODIUM SOY SAUCE

2 TABLESPOONS MINCED FRESH GINGER

1 TABLESPOON MINCED GARLIC

1 TABLESPOON SAVORY OIL (PAGE 81)

Freeze the tofu overnight, then thaw it in the package in the refrigerator or cold water. Squeeze out excess water and cut into 2-inch cubes.

Soak the noodles in the boiling water until soft, 8 to 10 minutes. Drain.

Divide the tofu, noodles, and sauce into 6 serving bowls. Arrange the vegetables on a large serving plate.

Make the broth: Bring all the broth ingredients to a boil in a large pot over high heat. Carefully transfer the pot to a hot plate on the table, or pour the hot broth into an electric wok or a metal fondue pot over a lit burner adjusted to the highest setting. If you don't have a large pot, add broth as the meal progresses.

Once the broth is boiling, each person, using a large slotted spoon or chopsticks, selects the hot pot ingredients he wants to cook and places them in the central cooking pot. Scald a few ingredients at a time for about 1 minute (tofu takes a little longer), eating and dipping as the food is cooked. Do not overcook.

Toward the end, divide up and enjoy the well-seasoned broth.

Makes 6 servings

TIPS

IF YOU ARE PRESSED FOR TIME OR DON'T HAVE THE EQUIPMENT, COMBINE ALL THE BROTH INGREDIENTS IN A LARGE POT AND BRING TO A BOIL. REDUCE HEAT TO MEDIUM-LOW. ADD TOFU, VEGETABLES, AND NOODLES, COVER, AND SIMMER FOR 4 TO 5 MINUTES, UNTIL VEGETABLES, AND NOODLES SOFTEN. GARNISH WITH 1 TABLESPOON SESAME OIL AND 2 MINCED GREEN ONIONS.

COMBINE THE SAUCE INGREDIENTS IN ONE LARGE BOWL; ADD ONE-THIRD OF THE SAUCE TO THE BROTH, THEN LADLE THE REST INTO SHALLOW BOWLS, ONE PER PERSON, AS A DIPPING SAUCE. SERVE HOT AND ENJOY.

Chicken Hot Pot Soup

Research conducted at the University of Nebraska Medical Center in Omaha has shown that a bowl of chicken soup is the best treatment for cold and flu. It is able to prevent inflammation and congestion and strengthens the immune system. When a cold causes you to have a stuffy nose, hot chilies such as jalapeños will help. They contain a compound called capsaicin, which will help you breathe easily again.

1 CUP SPICY HONEY-BASIL SAUCE (PAGE 94)

1 POUND SPINACH LEAVES

1 POUND BEAN SPROUTS

1 CUP 2-INCH WHITE ONION CUBES

4 GREEN ONIONS (WHITE AND GREEN PARTS), CUT INTO 2-INCH LENGTHS

½ POUND TENDER ASPARAGUS, CUT INTO 2-INCH LENGTHS

16 OUNCES FRESH OR FROZEN RAVIOLIS

½ POUND BONELESS, SKINLESS CHICKEN BREASTS, CUT INTO STRIPS

1 POUND FIRM FRESH TOFU

BROTH

5 CUPS GINSENG-CHICKEN STOCK (PAGE 69), MADE WITH AMERICAN GINSENG

2 CUPS SPRING WATER

3 CUPS FRESH OR FROZEN WHOLE-KERNEL CORN

SALT AND WHITE PEPPER TO TASTE

Divide the sauce into 6 serving bowls. Arrange the vegetables, raviolis, chicken, and tofu on serving plates.

Make the broth: Bring all the broth ingredients to a boil in a large pot over high heat. Carefully transfer the pot to a hot plate on the table, or pour the hot broth into an electric wok or a metal fondue pot over a lit burner adjusted to the highest setting. If you don't have a large pot, add broth and water as the meal progresses.

Once the broth is boiling, each person, using a large slotted spoon or chopsticks, selects the hot pot ingredients he or she wants to cook and places them in the central cooking pot. Scald a few ingredients at a time for about 1 minute (tofu takes a little longer), eating and dipping as the food is cooked. Do not overcook.

Toward the end, divide up and enjoy the well-seasoned soup with the dipping sauce.

Makes 6 servings (5 cups)

TIPS

IF YOU ARE PRESSED FOR TIME OR DON'T HAVE THE EQUIPMENT FOR HOT POT AT THE TABLE, COMBINE ALL THE BROTH INGREDIENTS IN A LARGE POT AND BRING TO A BOIL. REDUCE HEAT TO MEDIUM-LOW AND COVER. ADD TOFU, CHICKEN, AND RAVIOLI. SIMMER UNTIL RAVIOLIS ARE COOKED THROUGH, 8 TO 10 MINUTES (OR ACCORDING TO PACKAGE INSTRUCTIONS). ADD VEGETABLES AND COOK UNTIL HEATED THROUGH, ABOUT 2 MINUTES.

YOU MAY NEED TO ADD MORE WATER AS THE SOUP SIMMERS.

Meaty Hot Pot

This is a hearty stew, perfect for a winter day after a brisk walk. This traditional style of serving hot pot encourages the family to come together at the table. The key is to have all the ingredients ready to go, as you would for fondue.

½ POUND BEEF FLANK STEAK

¼ POUND BONELESS LEAN LAMB

½ POUND BONELESS, SKINLESS CHICKEN BREASTS, CUT INTO STRIPS

1 POUND FIRM TOFU

1 CUP 2-INCH WHITE ONION CUBES

4 GREEN ONIONS (WHITE AND GREEN PARTS), CUT INTO 2-INCH LENGTHS

½ POUND TENDER ASPARAGUS, CUT INTO 2-INCH LENGTHS

SAUCE

¼ CUP SOY SAUCE

¼ CUP RICE VINEGAR (PAGE 57)

2 TABLESPOONS OYSTER SAUCE

2 TABLESPOONS FRESH LEMON JUICE

¼ TEASPOON MINCED CHILI PEPPER

BROTH

5 CUPS GINSENG-CHICKEN STOCK (PAGE 69) OR CANNED CHICKEN STOCK

½ GINSENG ROOT OR 6 GINSENG SLICES

Prepare the beef and lamb by partially freezing it and then cutting it across the grain into very thin (⅛-inch) slices.

Arrange meat, tofu, and vegetables on serving plates.

Make the sauce: Combine the soy sauce, rice vinegar, oyster sauce, and lemon juice in a small bowl. Divide into 6 dipping bowls. Sprinkle a little of the chili pepper over each bowl.

Make the broth: Bring all the broth ingredients to a boil in a large pot over high heat. Carefully transfer the pot to a hot plate on the table, or pour the hot broth into an electric wok or a metal fondue pot over a lit burner adjusted to the highest setting. If you don't have a large pot, add broth and water as the meal progresses.

Once the broth is boiling, each person, using a large slotted spoon or chopsticks, selects the hot pot ingredients he or she wants to cook and places them in the central cooking pot. Scald a few ingredients at a time for about 1 minute (tofu takes a little longer), eating and dipping as the food is cooked. Do not overcook.

Toward the end, divide up and enjoy the well-seasoned soup with the dipping sauce.

Makes 6 servings

Hearty Mushroom–Tofu Soup

All you need to turn this soup into a satisfying meal is a simple salad and a loaf of fresh bread.

2 TABLESPOONS OLIVE OIL

1 POUND FRESH SHIITAKE MUSHROOMS, CAPS CUT INTO 2-INCH-WIDE STRIPS

4 QUARTER-SIZE SLICES FRESH GINGER

4 CUPS VEGETABLE AND MUSHROOM STOCK (PAGE 73)
   OR PURCHASED VEGETABLE STOCK

1 (12-OUNCE) PACKAGE FIRM SILKEN TOFU, CUT INTO ½-INCH CUBES

2 TABLESPOONS MISO

2 CUPS PACKED SPINACH LEAVES, COARSE STEMS REMOVED

2 TEASPOONS SESAME OIL

½ CUP CHOPPED GREEN ONIONS (WHITE AND GREEN PARTS)

SOY SAUCE TO TASTE

In a large saucepan, heat the oil over medium-high heat until hot. Add mushrooms and ginger and cook, stirring occasionally, until mushrooms are lightly browned, about 2 minutes.

Add the stock and bring to a boil. Add the tofu. Bring back to a boil. Reduce heat, cover, and simmer until tofu is heated through, 2 or 3 minutes.

Remove about ½ cup of the broth to a bowl. Add the miso and stir into a smooth, thin paste. Pour the paste back into the soup and add the spinach. Bring back to a boil. Remove from heat and ladle into bowls. Sprinkle with the sesame oil and green onions. Soy sauce may be passed at the table if desired. Serve hot.

Makes 4 servings

Hot and Sour Shrimp Soup

How hot this soup gets depends upon the type of chili you use. Your choice can range from mild poblano to hot-tempered habañero. I like the even-tempered jalapeños or Fresno chilies. This dish is a variation of a classic, well-known Thai seafood soup called tom yam gong. *It is a good soup to start a hot summer-day meal. Its sour, spicy, hot taste will perk up your appetite.*

4 CUPS GREEN TEA–SEAFOOD STOCK (PAGE 75)
    OR SPICY VEGETABLE STOCK (PAGE 71)

2 LEMONGRASS STALKS, BOTTOM 5 INCHES (PAGE 54)

1 FRESH RED CHILI, SEEDED AND CUT INTO THIN STRIPS

2 GARLIC CLOVES, CRUSHED

1 POUND RAW JUMBO SHRIMP, PEELED AND DEVEINED

1 CUP OYSTER MUSHROOMS, SLICED

2 TABLESPOONS FRESH LIME JUICE

1 TABLESPOON WATERCRESS LEAVES

4 GREEN ONIONS (WHITE PARTS ONLY), CHOPPED

THAI FISH SAUCE TO TASTE

FRESH CILANTRO LEAVES AND LIME SLICES,
    FOR GARNISH

Pour stock into a large pot. Add lemongrass, chili pepper, and garlic. Bring to a boil. Reduce the heat and simmer until fragrant, 3 to 4 minutes.

Add the shrimp, mushrooms, lime juice, and watercress leaves and bring to a second boil. Reduce the heat and cook until the

shrimp turn opaque, 3 to 4 minutes. Add the green onions. Season with fish sauce.

Garnish with lime slices and cilantro leaves. Serve hot.

Makes 4 to 6 servings (5 cups)

TIPS

DON'T OVERCOOK THE SHRIMP OR THEY WILL BECOME TOUGH.

FOR A VEGETARIAN VERSION, REPLACE THE SHRIMP WITH SLICES OF EXTRA-FIRM TOFU.

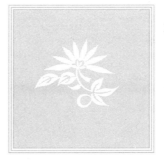

Lemongrass-Coconut-Flavored Tofu Soup

This aromatic soup is well balanced with coconut milk and tofu. It is full of ingredients with yin effect and ideal for summer. If you love strong-flavored spicy food, add more lemongrass and chili. Fish sauce is used in place of salt in this recipe. Season to your taste. Be creative. You can substitute meat and vegetables for the tofu.

4 CUPS GINSENG SEAFOOD STOCK (PAGE 77)
   OR CANNED CHICKEN STOCK

4 TABLESPOONS REDUCED-FAT, UNSWEETENED
   COCONUT MILK (PAGE 52)

6 PIECES FRESH OR DRIED GINSENG SLICES (ABOUT 0.3 OUNCE)

2 LEMONGRASS STALKS, BOTTOM 5 INCHES (PAGE 54)

½ CUP FROZEN WHOLE-KERNEL CORN

1 (3.5-OUNCE) PACKAGE FRESH ENOKI MUSHROOMS,
   BOTTOM PART DISCARDED

1 (16-OUNCE) BLOCK EXTRA-FIRM TOFU,
   CUT INTO 1-INCH CUBES

3 TABLESPOONS FRESH LEMON JUICE

FISH SAUCE TO TASTE

FOR GARNISH

2 GREEN ONIONS (WHITE PARTS ONLY), MINCED

2 TABLESPOONS EACH MINCED RED AND YELLOW BELL PEPPERS

CILANTRO OR MINT LEAVES

Place stock, coconut milk, ginseng, and lemongrass in a saucepan and bring to a boil. Reduce the heat; simmer for 3 minutes.

Add corn, mushrooms, and tofu. Bring to a second boil. Stir in the lemon juice and season with fish sauce.

Garnish with green onions, bell peppers, and cilantro leaves before serving.

Makes 6 servings (5 cups)

TIP

YOU CAN EAT THE GINSENG AT THE END; IT HAS A VERY STRONG FLAVOR.

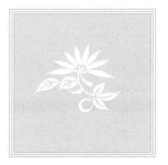

Curried Carrot and Apple Soup

This tasty and healthy soup is a great choice for entertaining. Its unusual ingredients and artistic presentation will please your guests' eyes as much as their appetites.

3 TABLESPOONS OLIVE OIL

2 TEASPOONS CURRY POWDER OR PASTE

2 TEASPOONS MINCED GINGER

1 POUND CARROTS, CHOPPED

1 LARGE ONION, CHOPPED INTO SMALL CUBES

1 GRANNY SMITH APPLE, PEELED AND CHOPPED INTO SMALL CUBES

2 CUPS SPICY VEGETABLE STOCK (PAGE 71)

1 CUP SOYMILK

SALT AND BLACK PEPPER TO TASTE

5 FRESH ASPARAGUS STALKS, BLANCHED, FOR GARNISH

2 TABLESPOONS PLAIN YOGURT, FOR GARNISH

Heat the oil in a large pot over medium heat. Add the curry powder and ginger and sauté until fragrant, about 30 seconds. Add the carrots, onion, and apple. Cover and cook over low heat until apple and carrots soften, about 10 minutes.

Spoon the carrot mixture into a food processor or blender and add the stock. Process until puréed.

Return the mixture to a saucepan. Stir in the soymilk and bring to a boil. Reduce heat and simmer for 5 minutes. Adjust the seasoning with salt and pepper. Pour into a large bowl. Create a five-leafed flower with the asparagus as the petals and the yogurt as the center.

Makes 4 servings (4 cups)

Tomato Crabmeat Egg Drop Soup

This soup makes a light meal on its own or served with Fresh Spring Rolls (page 122) or Seared Steak with Cucumber and Mango (page 117).

2 TABLESPOONS CANOLA OIL

2 CLOVES GARLIC, MINCED

1 GREEN ONION (WHITE AND GREEN PARTS), CHOPPED

3 FRESH OR DRIED SHIITAKE MUSHROOMS, CUT INTO 1-INCH CUBES

2 MEDIUM TOMATOES, CUT INTO 2-INCH CUBES

4 CUPS GINSENG SEAFOOD STOCK (PAGE 77) OR CANNED CHICKEN STOCK

1 CUP FRESH OR FROZEN CRABMEAT, OR IMITATION

1 EGG, WELL BEATEN

1 TEASPOON SESAME OIL

SALT AND WHITE PEPPER TO TASTE

CILANTRO LEAVES FOR GARNISH

Heat the oil in a large, heavy saucepan on medium high heat and sauté the garlic, onion, and mushrooms until fragrant, about 2 minutes. Add tomatoes, reduce the heat to medium low, stir, and cook for 2 to 3 minutes.

Stir in the stock and bring to a boil. Add crabmeat and bring to a second boil. Turn off heat. Slowly pour in the beaten egg, while stirring the soup in one direction with a chopstick or fork so the egg forms long threads.

Stir in sesame oil. Garnish with cilantro leaves. Serve hot.

Makes 4 to 6 servings (5 cups)

Seafood Pumpkin Pot

Every fall when I see so many pumpkins in stores, it always reminds me of a dish I ate in China made with winter melon. This pumpkin pot is inspired from that. Why not try it for your next Halloween party? As a plus the pumpkin is your serving vessel, which means one less dish to wash after the party.

1 MEDIUM BAKING PUMPKIN (8 TO 10 POUNDS)

2 TABLESPOONS EXTRA-VIRGIN OLIVE OIL

1 POUND SMALL WHITE ONIONS, CUT INTO ½-INCH CHUNKS

½ POUND LARGE RAW SHRIMP, PEELED AND DEVEINED

½ POUND SEA SCALLOPS

5 CUPS GREEN TEA–SEAFOOD STOCK (PAGE 75)

3 CUPS WATER

4 PIECES GINSENG, SLICED (OPTIONAL)

1 MEDIUM ZUCCHINI, CUT INTO 1-INCH CHUNKS

6 FRESH OR DRIED SHIITAKE MUSHROOMS

½ CUP FRESH OR FROZEN CRABMEAT

1 MEDIUM YELLOW SQUASH, CUT INTO 1-INCH CHUNKS

SALT AND BLACK PEPPER TO TASTE

6 SPRIGS CILANTRO, OR 8 PIECES BASIL

Select an attractive, unblemished pumpkin. Rinse and dry the outside with a kitchen towel. Cut an approximate 2-inch circular hole into top of pumpkin. Scoop out the seeds and membranes. Carve a decorative motif on the skin around the sides, and use a sharp knife to make zigzag cuts around the rim.

In a large pot, heat the oil over medium-high heat until hot. Add the onions and cook until golden. Add the shrimp and scallops and stir-fry until they are opaque, 1 to 2 minutes. Add the stock,

water, ginseng, zucchini, and mushrooms and bring to a boil. Reduce the heat to low, cover, and simmer for 5 minutes.

Place pumpkin shell upright in a heatproof dish and put on a rack in a steamer. Pour in boiling soup. Add crabmeat and squash. Cover and steam over briskly boiling water until the pumpkin meat softens, 20 to 30 minutes. Season with salt and pepper.

Garnish with cilantro. To serve, spoon out stew, scooping some pumpkin meat with each serving.

Makes 6 servings

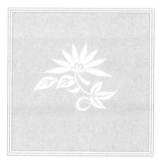

Soup of Harmony

This dish is a real eye catcher. It presents another delicious way to enjoy beans. Serve it as thick soup or as dip for chips and vegetables.

1 (15-OUNCE) CAN GARBANZO BEANS

2 CUPS BREWED GINSENG TEA (SEE PAGE 35)
   OR GREEN TEA (SEE PAGE 39)

2 GARLIC CLOVES, MINCED

1 TABLESPOON FRESH LEMON JUICE

3 TABLESPOONS OLIVE OIL

1 (15-OUNCE) CAN BLACK (TURTLE) BEANS

1 JALAPEÑO CHILI PEPPER, SEEDED AND CHOPPED

2 GREEN ONIONS (WHITE AND GREEN PARTS), FINELY CHOPPED

SALT AND BLACK PEPPER TO TASTE

Drain the garbanzo beans. Reserve 3 beans for garnish. Place the remaining beans, 1 cup of the tea, garlic, lemon juice, and 1½ tablespoons of the olive oil in a food processor or blender. Process until puréed and transfer to a large measuring cup or container with a pouring spout.

Drain the black beans. Reserve 3 beans for garnish. Place the remaining beans, 1 cup of the tea, 1½ tablespoons of the olive oil, chili, and green onions in a food processor or blender. Process until puréed and transfer to a large measuring cup or container with a pouring spout. (Add a little vegetable stock or water if the soup is too thick.)

Season both purée bean mixtures with salt and pepper. Slowly pour the soups simultaneously into the opposite sides of a large serving bowl. Use a spoon to gently push the edge of the black bean to form an *S* shape. The result should resemble the yin and yang symbol. Garnish with reserved black beans placed at the center of the garbanzo purée and garbanzo beans in the center of the black bean purée.

Makes 6 servings (4 cups)

LONGEVITY AND GINSENG

MANY OF THE CHINESE LEADERS, SUCH AS MAO ZEDONG AND DENG XIAOPING, LIVED LONG LIVES DESPITE THEIR CONSTANT BRUTAL POWER STRUGGLES. ONE OF THEIR SECRETS FOR LONGEVITY WAS TAKING THE FINEST MANCHURIAN GINSENG ROOT. THIS GINSENG PLANT WAS CULTIVATED FROM THE BEST WILD STOCK IN THE NORTHERN MOUNTAINS AND WAS FIRST PLANTED DURING THE MING DYNASTY OVER FOUR HUNDRED YEARS AGO. WORD HAS IT THAT CHINESE LEADERS BEGIN THEIR CONFERENCES BY PASSING AROUND TRAYS FILLED WITH GINSENG.

Italian Seafood Stew

Many times I'm asked, "Do you cook only Asian food?" The question made me think about my daily cooking. Many of my dishes are no longer traditionally Asian, but almost always I either include Asian ingredients or use Asian cooking methods. I guess it is fair to say that I cook in an Asian fusion style.

This seafood stew is cooling.

6 SMALL NEW POTATOES, PEELED AND QUARTERED

2 SMALL YELLOW ZUCCHINI, CUT INTO BITE-SIZE CHUNKS

2 TABLESPOONS OLIVE OIL

4 GARLIC CLOVES, CRUSHED

1 MEDIUM RED ONION, CUT INTO 1-INCH CHUNKS

1½ CUPS GREEN TEA–SEAFOOD STOCK (PAGE 75) OR VEGETABLE AND MUSHROOM STOCK (PAGE 73)

8 LARGE MUSSELS, SCRUBBED AND DEBEARDED

½ POUND MEDIUM SHRIMP, PEELED AND DEVEINED

½ POUND MEDIUM SCALLOPS

½ CUP TOMATO JUICE OR PASTE

½ CUP RED WINE

1 TEASPOON SUGAR

SALT AND WHITE PEPPER TO TASTE

2 TABLESPOONS CHOPPED FRESH OR DRIED BASIL LEAVES

In a large saucepan, bring 4 cups water to a boil. Add the potatoes and cook until almost tender, about 10 minutes. Add the zucchini and cook until just tender, about 5 minutes. Drain and set aside.

In a large Dutch oven or heavy soup pot, heat the olive oil over medium heat until hot. Add the garlic and onion and sauté, stirring frequently, until onion is tender, about 3 minutes. Add the stock,

mussels, shrimp, and scallops. Simmer, stirring occasionally, until mussels open and shrimp turn opaque.

Add the tomato juice, wine, and sugar. Season with salt and pepper. Stir in potato and zucchini; bring to a boil. Garnish with basil.

Makes 4 servings

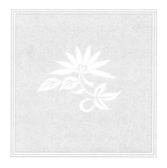

Creamy Fresh Pea Soup

This light, cooling soup is ideal for summer outings. Serve it with crusty bread or wrappers for a satisfying lunch.

2 TABLESPOONS BUTTER

4 CLOVES GARLIC, MINCED

1 SMALL ONION, FINELY CHOPPED

3 CUPS BREWED GREEN TEA (SEE PAGE 39)

1 CUP SOYMILK

3 CUPS FRESH OR THAWED FROZEN GREEN PEAS

SALT AND WHITE PEPPER TO TASTE

¼ CUP PLAIN YOGURT

2 TABLESPOONS FRESH MINT LEAVES, MINCED

Melt the butter in a large saucepan. Add the garlic and onion and sauté until onion is softened, about 3 minutes.

Stir in tea and soymilk and bring to a boil. Reduce the heat, add the peas, cover, and simmer for 10 minutes.

Transfer the soup to a blender or food processor. Process until puréed. Return the soup to the saucepan and heat thoroughly. Season with salt and pepper. Serve lukewarm or chilled. Garnish each serving with a dollop of yogurt and sprinkle with mint.

Makes 5 or 6 servings

Shrimp Wontons with Shiitake Mushroom–Miso Soup

All you need to turn this hearty soup into a satisfying meal is a simple salad. Try serving with Tea-Crusted Tofu over Greens (page 176) or Thai-Style Cabbage Salad (page 181).

BROTH

6 CUPS BOILING WATER

1 GREEN TEA BAG OR 1 TABLESPOON LOOSE GREEN TEA

3 TABLESPOONS RED MISO (SOYBEAN PASTE) OR TAHINI

1 CUP THINLY SLICED SHIITAKE MUSHROOM CAPS (ABOUT 3 OUNCES)

FILLING

$1/3$ CUP MINCED GREEN ONIONS (WHITE AND GREEN PARTS)

1 TABLESPOON LOW-SODIUM SOY SAUCE

2 TEASPOONS RICE VINEGAR

2 TEASPOONS DARK SESAME OIL

2 TEASPOONS GRATED PEELED FRESH GINGER

$1/8$ TEASPOON WHITE PEPPER

$1/2$ POUND LARGE SHRIMP, PEELED AND FINELY CHOPPED

$1/4$ POUND LEAN GROUND PORK

2 GARLIC CLOVES, MINCED

20 WONTON WRAPPERS OR GYOZA SKINS (SEE PAGE 53)

$1/4$ CUP THINLY SLICED RED BELL PEPPER

2 TABLESPOONS SLICED GREEN ONIONS

To prepare broth, pour the boiling water over tea bag in a large saucepan; steep for 5 minutes. Remove and reserve tea bag. Bring tea mixture to a boil. Add miso, stirring with a whisk until blended. Add mushroom caps; bring to a boil. Reduce heat and simmer 5 minutes. Remove from heat; cover and set aside.

To prepare filling, cut open reserved tea bag and pour out loose tea; chop, if needed. Combine loose tea and filling ingredients in a medium bowl. Working with one wonton wrapper at a time (cover remaining wrappers with a damp towel to keep them from drying out), spoon 1 tablespoon of the filling mixture on half of each wrapper. Moisten the edges of wrapper with water; bring the 2 opposite corners together. Pinch edges together to seal, forming a triangle.

Bring reserved tea mixture to a boil; add wontons, gently stir, and cook 4 minutes or until wontons float to the top. Ladle 5 wontons and 1 cup broth into each of 4 bowls. Divide bell pepper and onion slices evenly among bowls. Serve immediately.

Makes 4 servings

TIP

WONTONS FREEZE VERY WELL. TO FREEZE: FIRST, PLACE THEM ON A LIGHTLY FLOURED PLATE SO THEY DON'T TOUCH. PUT THE PLATE IN YOUR FREEZER UNTIL THE WONTONS ARE FROZEN SOLID. THEN REMOVE THEM FROM THE PLATE AND SEAL THEM IN A PLASTIC FREEZER BAG. DROP THE FROZEN WONTONS INTO BOILING SOUP AND COOK THEM A LITTLE LONGER THAN FRESH ONES.

Red Soup with Watercress

This colorful, delicious soup is beautiful and cheerful. It was inspired by one of the soups I ate in a Russian restaurant in Beijing.

1½ TABLESPOONS BUTTER

3 CLOVES GARLIC, CHOPPED

1 SMALL RED CAYENNE PEPPER, SEEDED AND CHOPPED

4 RED BELL PEPPERS, CHOPPED

2 SMALL LEEKS (WHITE PART ONLY)

¼ CUP CHOPPED TOMATO

3 CUPS GREEN TEA–SEAFOOD STOCK (PAGE 75)
    OR GINSENG-SEAFOOD STOCK (PAGE 77)

1 TEASPOON FRESH LEMON JUICE

SALT TO TASTE

3 TABLESPOONS WATERCRESS LEAVES

Melt the butter in a saucepan over medium heat. Add the garlic and cayenne pepper and sauté until fragrant. Add the bell peppers and leeks and sauté, stirring occasionally, until soft.

Stir in the tomato and half of the stock, and bring to a boil. Transfer the mixture to a food processor or blender and process until puréed. Return to the pan and add the rest of the stock. Stir in the lemon juice and season with salt. Bring to a boil.

Ladle into serving bowls. Garnish with watercress leaves.

Makes 4 to 6 servings

Chicken Stew

Use natural chicken that is hormone- and antibiotic-free if you can. At some health food stores, you can even find chicken raised on a vegetarian diet. You will find that these meats are not only healthy but taste so much better. If you are pressed for time, ask the meat department to cut up the chicken for you.

3 TABLESPOONS BUTTER

3 GARLIC CLOVES, CHOPPED

¾ POUND BONELESS, SKINLESS CHICKEN BREAST, CUT INTO 2-INCH CHUNKS

3 MEDIUM CARROTS, PEELED AND CUT INTO 2-INCH CHUNKS

2 YELLOW SQUASH, CUT INTO 2-INCH CHUNKS

2 MEDIUM CELERY STALKS, CUT INTO 2-INCH-WIDE STRIPS

1 CUP FRESH SHIITAKE MUSHROOMS, CUT INTO 2-INCH-WIDE STRIPS

¼ CUP RED WINE

3 CUPS VEGETABLE AND MUSHROOM STOCK (PAGE 73)

SALT AND BLACK PEPPER TO TASTE

1½ TABLESPOONS DRIED BASIL LEAVES

In a nonstick cooking pan, melt 2 tablespoons of the butter. Add garlic and sauté until brown, about 1 minute. Add the chicken and cook until golden brown. Place in a bowl and set aside.

Heat the remaining 1 tablespoon butter in the pan. Add the carrots, squash, celery, and mushrooms and sauté until soft. Stir in the wine and cook 1 minute. Stir in stock and bring to a boil. Reduce heat to low, cover, and simmer until vegetables are tender, 20 to 25 minutes. Season with salt and pepper. Garnish with basil leaves. Serve hot.

Makes 4 to 6 servings

Essential Miso Soup with Tofu and Noodles

Fresh udon noodles work best for this dish, but if you can't find them, any fresh linguine or wide rice noodles will do. This soup makes a great light lunch.

½ POUND NOODLES, UDON OR SOBA

4 CUPS VEGETABLE AND MUSHROOM STOCK (PAGE 73) OR WATER

2 TABLESPOONS MISO

8 OUNCES FLAVORED BAKED TOFU (PACKAGED, OR RECIPE ON PAGE 125),
    CUT INTO ½-INCH CUBES

½ CUP PEELED, THINLY SLICED CARROTS

3 GREEN ONIONS (WHITE AND GREEN PARTS), THINLY SLICED

1 TABLESPOON SESAME OIL

¼ CUP BEAN SPROUTS

LOW-SODIUM SOY SAUCE TO TASTE

Cook the noodles according to the package directions. Rinse under cold water. Drain and set aside.

In a soup pot, bring the stock to a boil. In a small bowl, mash the miso with about ¼ cup warm stock until it forms a smooth sauce; then stir the miso sauce back into the soup.

Add the tofu, cooked noodles, and carrots. Bring the soup back to a boil. Reduce the heat to low and simmer for 3 minutes.

Stir in the green onions and sesame oil. Top with sprouts. Season with soy sauce, if desired. Serve hot.

Makes 4 servings

Crabmeat, Corn, and Bean Soup

Beans are an easy, convenient, and economical way of getting protein. If you have time, soak the beans in water overnight before cooking; otherwise, use canned or frozen beans.

2 TABLESPOONS BUTTER

6 OUNCES FRESH OR CANNED CRABMEAT,
    DRAINED AND FLAKED

4 CUPS WATER

1 TABLESPOON MINCED FRESH GINGER

½ POUND DRIED BLACK-EYED PEAS

1 CUP FRESH OR FROZEN WHOLE-KERNEL CORN

1 CUP FRESH SUNFLOWER SPROUTS

SALT AND WHITE PEPPER TO TASTE

Melt the butter in a cooking pot. Add the crabmeat and sauté for 1 minute. Add the water, ginger, and black-eyed peas. Bring to a boil. Reduce the heat, cover the pan, and simmer, stirring occasionally, until black-eyed peas are tender, 20 to 25 minutes.

Add the corn and bean sprouts and bring to a boil. Season with salt and pepper. Serve hot.

Makes 4 servings

Vegetarian Chowder

The name chowder originated from a French word, chaudière. *It refers to the "supper in a large pot made from the leftovers from the fishermen's sale of their daily catch." I experimented with replacing the seafood with soy and had this great result.*

2 TABLESPOONS BUTTER

1 SMALL ONION, CHOPPED

2 CUPS WHOLE-KERNEL CORN

½ CUP FRESH SHIITAKE MUSHROOMS CAPS, MINCED

2½ CUPS SOYMILK

1 (16-OUNCE) BLOCK FIRM TOFU, DRAINED,
    CUT INTO ½-INCH CUBES

1 CUP SOY CREAMER OR WHOLE MILK

2 GREEN ONIONS, MINCED

½ TEASPOON DRIED CHILI PEPPER (OPTIONAL)

SALT AND BLACK PEPPER TO TASTE

In a nonstick cooking pan over medium heat, melt the butter. Add the onion and sauté until softened, about 4 minutes.

Add the corn and mushrooms. Sauté for 1 minute. Add the soymilk and bring to a boil. Reduce the heat; add the tofu. Cover the pan and simmer, stirring occasionally, for 3 minutes.

Add the creamer. Bring to a rapid boil. Stir in the green onions and chili pepper, if using, and season with salt and pepper. Serve hot.

Makes 4 servings

6. Dinners in a Minute: Salads

As with tea and ginseng, the Chinese divide food into categories. There are cooling, neutral, and warming foods. See page 7. Cooling foods are yin: soothing and mild. Warming foods are yang: invigorating, spicy, and high in protein. Neutral foods provide a balance between the two. By combining cooling vegetables with warming spices, meats, and nuts, enhanced by the right kind of ginseng, you get a well-balanced meal with delicious tastes and therapeutic effects.

It is interesting that the modern health findings and the USDA Food Pyramid agree with the ancient Chinese medical text *The Yellow Emperor's Classic of Internal Medicine*, compiled about the fourth century B.C. It states, "One should have grains and cereals for body growth; vegetables and fruit for supplement and assistance; meat and protein for nutrition."

Salads have been trendy in the West for years, but it's not a traditional or popular way for Asians to eat their vegetables. This is partly due to unsafe tap water. In many parts of Asia, even in the major cities, it is not safe to consume tap water without boiling it first. This is why most vegetable dishes are cooked. After I came to the United States, I delighted in the many varieties of salad, especially with the growing availability of organic vegetables.

A salad is a quick and easy way to prepare a nutritious meal. With the combination of vegetables, rice, pasta, or potato, topped with meat, tofu, nuts, or seafood, you have vitamins, carbohydrates, and protein. Many of the recipes in this chapter can be served as a whole meal in themselves.

DIFFERENT TYPES OF VEGETARIANS

VEGETARIAN: DOES NOT EAT MEAT, POULTRY, OR FISH. EATS GRAINS, NUTS, SEEDS, VEGETABLES, AND FRUITS WITH OR WITHOUT THE USE OF DAIRY PRODUCTS AND EGGS.

VEGAN: DOES NOT EAT ANIMAL FLESH, DAIRY PRODUCTS, EGGS, OR ANY OTHER ANIMAL PRODUCT.

FRUITARIAN: VEGAN DIET IN WHICH VERY FEW PROCESSED OR COOKED FOODS ARE EATEN. CONSISTS MAINLY OF RAW FRUIT, GRAINS, AND NUTS. FOLLOWERS EAT ONLY FOODS THAT DON'T KILL THE PLANT. (APPLES AND SQUASH CAN BE PICKED WITHOUT KILLING THE PLANT; CARROTS CANNOT.)

LACTO-OVO: EATS BOTH DAIRY PRODUCTS AND EGGS BUT NO MEAT, POULTRY, OR FISH. THIS IS THE MOST COMMON TYPE OF VEGETARIAN DIET IN THE UNITED STATES.

LACTO: AVOIDS MEAT, POULTRY, FISH, AND EGGS BUT EATS DAIRY PRODUCTS.

OVO: AVOIDS MEAT, POULTRY, FISH, AND DAIRY PRODUCTS BUT EATS EGGS.

MACROBIOTIC: A USUALLY VEGAN DIET OF ALMOST EXCLUSIVELY COOKED FOODS WITH A HEAVY EMPHASIS ON WHOLE GRAINS AND VEGETABLES; SOME FOLLOWERS EAT FISH.

PESCETARIAN/PESCO: EATS PLANT PRODUCTS AND FISH.

Garden Salad with Shrimp and Ginger-Sesame Dressing

Served with fresh, crusty bread, this salad is great for a picnic. You can replace the shrimp with scallops or grilled salmon. Wash only the portion of the bell peppers you are going to use. The leftover halves will keep longer in the refrigerator if unwashed and wrapped in a paper towel to absorb the moisture.

GINGER-SESAME DRESSING

1 TABLESPOON BUTTER

2 SMALL CLOVES GARLIC, MINCED

1 TABLESPOON GRATED FRESH GINGER

½ CUP WHIPPING CREAM

1 TABLESPOON FRESH LEMON JUICE

2 TABLESPOONS MINCED CILANTRO OR BASIL LEAVES

SALT AND WHITE PEPPER TO TASTE

1 MEDIUM CARROT

4-OUNCE BAG BABY GREEN SALAD MIX

½ SMALL RED BELL PEPPER, CUT INTO MATCHSTICK-SIZE PIECES

½ SMALL YELLOW BELL PEPPER, CUT INTO MATCHSTICK-SIZE PIECES

2 TABLESPOONS CANOLA OIL

2 TABLESPOONS BLACK SESAME SEEDS

1 TABLESPOON THINLY SHREDDED GINGER

2 TEASPOONS MINCED FRESH RED CAYENNE CHILI PEPPER

1 POUND RAW LARGE SHRIMP, PEELED AND DEVEINED

1 TABLESPOON FISH SAUCE

½ TABLESPOON COOKING WINE OR SAKE

Make the dressing: Melt butter in a small saucepan over medium-high heat. Add the garlic and ginger and sauté until lightly browned, about 1 minute. Add the cream and bring to a rapid boil. Remove from heat. Stir in the lemon juice and cilantro. Season with salt and pepper. Makes ¾ cup.

Wash and peel the carrot. Cut diagonally into thin slices, then cut lengthwise into matchstick-size pieces. Toss together the salad mix, bell peppers, and carrot in a large serving bowl.

Heat the oil in a medium nonstick cooking pan over medium-high heat. Add the sesame seeds, ginger, and chili and sauté until fragrant, about 30 seconds. Add the shrimp and stir-fry for 1 minute. Stir in fish sauce and wine. Stir-fry until shrimp are opaque, about 1 minute.

Pour dressing over salad and toss. Top with the shrimp mixture.

Makes 4 to 6 servings

Shrimp Noodle Salad

Not your typical noodle salad! The sauce adds a tangy touch to the shrimp and noodles.

3 CUPS SPRING WATER

3 GINSENG TEA BAGS

5 OUNCES DRY BEAN THREAD NOODLES (PAGE 55)

½ POUND PEELED, COOKED MEDIUM SHRIMP

4 OUNCES SNOW PEAS, TRIMMED AND CUT INTO 2-INCH STRIPS

1 SMALL RED BELL PEPPER, CUT INTO 2-INCH STRIPS

4 GREEN ONIONS (WHITE PART ONLY), CUT INTO 2-INCH STRIPS

SALT AND WHITE PEPPER TO TASTE

1 CUP SPICY HONEY-BASIL SAUCE (PAGE 94)

¼ CUP BASIL LEAVES, FOR GARNISH

In a big pot, bring the water to a boil and add the tea bags and noodles. Turn off heat, cover, and let noodles soak until softened, about 5 minutes. Drain, rinse under cold water, and drain thoroughly.

In a large salad bowl, combine the noodles with shrimp, snow peas, bell pepper, and green onions. Season with salt and pepper. Toss with the sauce. Garnish with basil leaves and serve.

Makes 4 servings

Shrimp-Mango Salad

This one was inspired by a salad I ate at a beach resort in Thailand. I wrote down the ingredients on a napkin as I ate the meal and developed this recipe soon after I returned home.

½ POUND RAW SHRIMP, PEELED AND DEVEINED

¼ CUP THAI SAUCE (PAGE 91)

2 TABLESPOONS OLIVE OIL

4 CLOVES GARLIC, CHOPPED

1 CUP SUGAR SNAP PEAS

2 GREEN ONIONS (GREEN AND WHITE PARTS),
    CUT INTO 2-INCH LENGTHS

2 CUP MIXED SALAD LEAVES

2 MANGOES, SLICED

¼ CUP CANDIED NUTS (PAGE 102)

In a bowl, mix the shrimp and sauce together. Cover and refrigerate for 15 minutes or longer.

Heat oil in a nonstick cooking pan. Add the garlic and sauté until fragrant. Add the shrimp and stir-fry until shrimp turn opaque throughout, about 3 minutes. Add the peas and green onions. Stir-fry until peas turn bright green and green onions begin to soften.

To serve, arrange the salad leaves on one side of 4 large plates, and mango slices on the other side, in a fan shape. Spoon the shrimp mixture onto salad leaves. Top with the nuts.

Makes 4 servings

Shrimp Pasta Salad

I always keep a bag of peeled, raw shrimp in my freezer. It's a great way to add a quick protein boost to a dish. Frozen cooked shrimp tends to have less flavor than the uncooked, but they do save you time. This dish is another good example of using Asian ingredients the western way.

½ POUND RAW SHRIMP, PEELED AND DEVEINED

½ CUP GREEN CHILI SAUCE (PAGE 92)

12 OUNCES BOW TIE PASTA

2 TABLESPOONS OLIVE OIL

4 CLOVES GARLIC, CHOPPED

½ CUP SLICED FRESH SHIITAKE MUSHROOM CAPS

½ CUP OIL-PACKED, SUN-DRIED TOMATOES, DRAINED AND SLICED

2 TABLESPOONS CHOPPED FRESH CHIVES

3 TABLESPOONS FRESHLY GRATED PARMESAN CHEESE

In a bowl, mix the shrimp and sauce together. Cover and refrigerate for 15 minutes or longer.

Cook the pasta according to package directions. Drain, rinse in cold water, and place the pasta in a salad bowl.

Heat oil in a nonstick cooking pan over medium heat. Add the garlic and sauté until fragrant. Add the shrimp and sauce and stir-fry until shrimp turn opaque throughout, 2 to 3 minutes. Stir in the mushrooms and sun-dried tomatoes. Stir-fry until the mushrooms heat through, about 2 minutes.

Toss the shrimp mixture with the pasta and garnish with chives and cheese.

Makes 4 servings

Noodle and Smoked Salmon Salad

Almost every Asian country has its own variety of the cold noodle salad. This creation combines those from a few Asian countries.

½ POUND THIN NOODLES

2 TEASPOONS ASIAN SESAME OIL

3 GREEN ONIONS (GREEN AND WHITE PARTS),
    CUT INTO 2-INCH LENGTHS

4 SPRIGS FRESH CILANTRO, CUT INTO 2-INCH LENGTHS

4 OUNCES SOYBEAN SPROUTS

¼ CUP ZANTE CURRANTS

½ CUP ½-INCH CUBES SMOKED SALMON

1 CUP THAI SAUCE (PAGE 91)

2 LARGE TOMATOES, THINLY SLICED

Cook the noodles according to the package directions. Drain and rinse under cold water.

In a large bowl, toss the noodles, sesame oil, green onions, cilantro, sprouts, currants, and smoked salmon with the sauce.

Arrange the tomato slices on a serving plate. Pile the noodle mixture on top of the sliced tomatoes and serve cold.

Makes 4 servings

Cherry Tomato Tuna Salad

This multicolored salad's delicious taste is matched by its great eye appeal. I like to serve it in a terra-cotta–colored bowl.

½ POUND CHERRY TOMATOES, HALVED

½ POUND RADISHES, CUT INTO 1-INCH CUBES

1 MEDIUM CUCUMBER, CUT INTO 1-INCH CUBES

2 CELERY RIBS, CUT INTO 1-INCH CUBES

1 CUP WHITE WINE SAUCE (PAGE 87)

2 (7-OUNCE) CANS TUNA, DRAINED AND FLAKED

4 RED LETTUCE LEAVES

4 GREEN LETTUCE LEAVES

2 GREEN ONIONS (GREEN AND WHITE PARTS), MINCED

Place the tomato, radishes, cucumber, and celery in a big salad bowl. Add the sauce and toss to coat.

Add the tuna. Toss gently until well mixed.

Arrange the lettuce leaves, alternating red and green, on a plate. Spoon the salad into the center. Garnish with the green onions.

Makes 4 to 6 servings

Fennel-Orange-Apple Salad

The licorice flavor of fennel combines nicely with the sweet orange and crunchy apple.

2 MEDIUM FENNEL BULBS

2 SWEET ORANGES

2 FIRM APPLES

1 TEASPOON FRESH LEMON JUICE

4 OUNCES FETA CHEESE, CRUMBLED

¼ CUP APPLE-ORANGE SAUCE (PAGE 98)

¼ CUP PARSLEY LEAVES, CHOPPED

Wash fennel bulbs and cut them in half lengthwise. Trim green outer leaves. Thinly slice fennel crosswise. Place it in a salad bowl.

Peel the oranges; remove white pith and membrane. Cut into segments, holding over a bowl. Arrange over the fennel; add any juice from the oranges.

Peel the apples, core, and thinly slice. Sprinkle with the lemon juice. Toss with the fennel, oranges, and cheese. Spoon the sauce over the salad and toss to combine. Garnish with the parsley.

Makes 4 servings

Wild Rice with Dried Cherries and Pine Nuts

This is a good way to use up leftover rice. Toast the nuts ahead of time. They will keep for up to a week in an airtight container in the refrigerator.

1 CUP WILD RICE

½ CUP BROWN RICE

3 CUPS COLD WATER

¼ CUP DRIED CHERRIES

3 GREEN ONIONS (GREEN AND WHITE PARTS),
    CUT INTO ½-INCH LENGTHS

2 TABLESPOONS FRESH CILANTRO LEAVES

1 TABLESPOON MINCED FRESH GINGER

¾ CUP ORANGE AND SOY SAUCE (PAGE 89)

¼ CUP PINE NUTS, TOASTED (SEE TIP, PAGE 96)

SALT AND BLACK PEPPER TO TASTE

Rinse the rice thoroughly with cold water. Place the rice in a 6-quart saucepan; add the water. Bring the rice to a boil. Reduce heat to medium-low and let simmer covered until rice has puffed up and most of the liquid is absorbed, 45 to 50 minutes. Cool slightly.

In a big salad bowl, mix the rice, cherries, green onions, cilantro leaves, and ginger. Pour the sauce over the salad and mix well. Just before serving, toss in the toasted nuts and season to taste.

Makes 4 servings

Tea-Crusted Tofu over Greens

To me, green tea and tofu seem to go hand in hand; green tea's delicate flavor beautifully complements tofu's smoothness. A light honey-vinegar dressing rounds out this dish. It's one of my favorites.

VINAIGRETTE

2 TEASPOONS LOOSE GREEN TEA OR 2 GREEN TEA BAGS

½ CUP BOILING SPRING WATER

1 TABLESPOON HONEY

1 TABLESPOON RICE VINEGAR

½ TABLESPOON FISH SAUCE

2 CLOVES GARLIC, CHOPPED

1 GREEN ONION, MINCED

1 (16-OUNCE) BLOCK EXTRA-FIRM TOFU

2 TABLESPOONS OLIVE OIL

2 TEASPOONS LOOSE GREEN TEA OR CONTENTS OF 2 TEA BAGS

1½ TABLESPOONS WHITE SESAME SEEDS

⅛ TEASPOON SALT

4 CUPS BABY GREENS SALAD MIX

2 ASIAN PEARS OR BOSC PEARS, CUBED

1 CUP HALVED CHERRY TOMATOES (ABOUT 8 OUNCES)

½ CUP CANDIED NUTS (PAGE 102)

Make the vinaigrette: Place the tea in a teacup and pour in the boiling water. Cover and let brew for 2 to 3 minutes. Save the brewed tea for the dressing and discard the tea leaves.

Combine the tea and remaining dressing ingredients in a bowl and mix well. Cover and refrigerate for at least 30 minutes before using. Makes about ½ cup.

Place the tofu on a flat surface and press out the water. Dry with paper towels. Cut the tofu into 8 equal cubes by first cutting the block into 2 sheets, then cutting both sheets in half and then in quarters.

Heat a nonstick wok or large frying pan over medium-high heat. Add the oil and swirl to coat. Add the tea leaves, sesame seeds, and salt and sauté till fragrant. Place the tofu slices on top and pan-fry until golden brown, about 3 minutes. Turn the tofu and pan-fry the other side until golden brown, about 3 minutes. Drain the tofu on paper towels. Cut to desired size.

Toss together salad greens, pears, and tomatoes in a salad bowl. Arrange the tofu slices over the salad, spoon the dressing on top, top with the nuts, and serve.

Makes 4 servings

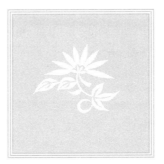

Garden Salad with Feta Cheese

The first time I ate feta, I was shocked by its strong flavor. But its smell reminds me of a type of fermented tofu sold on the streets of my hometown, Wuhan, nicknamed "stinky tofu." You can smell the vendors that sell it even if they are blocks away.

2 TABLESPOONS OLIVE OIL

1 TABLESPOON FRESH LEMON JUICE

3 CLOVES GARLIC, MINCED

2 TABLESPOONS CHOPPED FRESH MINT

4 CUPS BABY GREEN SALAD MIX

½ RED ONION, THINLY SLICED

FRESHLY GROUND PEPPER TO TASTE

4 OUNCES FETA CHEESE, CRUMBLED

12 PITTED BLACK OLIVES

In a small bowl, combine the oil, lemon juice, garlic, and mint. Mix well and set aside.

In a large salad bowl, mix salad greens and red onion. Pour dressing over salad and toss. Season with pepper.

Arrange salad on 4 serving plates. Top with feta cheese and olives.

Makes 4 servings

VARIATION
REPLACE THE CHEESE WITH CUBED TOFU.

Spinach Salad with Avocado and Tofu

The sharp taste of the parsley in this salad is a perfect complement to the sweet ripe avocados and chilled tofu. Served with a good bread, this tasty and beautiful salad makes a great lunch.

1 (12-OUNCE) PACKAGE REDUCED-FAT, EXTRA-FIRM SILKEN TOFU,
    DRAINED AND CUT INTO $\frac{1}{2}$-INCH CUBES

3 TABLESPOONS EAST MEETS WEST SAUCE (PAGE 82)

SPICY GARLIC DRESSING

$\frac{1}{2}$ FRESH RED CHILI PEPPER, MINCED

1 TABLESPOON MINCED LEMON PEEL

2 CLOVES GARLIC, FINELY MINCED

2 TABLESPOONS LOOSE GREEN TEA LEAVES

2 TABLESPOONS EXTRA-VIRGIN OLIVE OIL

$\frac{1}{2}$ TABLESPOON RED VINEGAR

1 TABLESPOON FRESH LEMON JUICE

$\frac{1}{8}$ TEASPOON SALT

$\frac{1}{4}$ TEASPOON BLACK PEPPER

2 CUPS BABY SPINACH LEAVES, LARGE STEMS REMOVED

$\frac{1}{2}$ CUP TIGHTLY PACKED PARSLEY LEAVES, CLEANED,
    DRIED, AND CHOPPED

1 AVOCADO, CUBED

$\frac{1}{4}$ CUP PINE NUTS, TOASTED (SEE TIP, PAGE 96),
    OR CANDIED NUTS (PAGE 102)

In a medium bowl, combine the tofu and sauce. Cover and refrigerate for 1 hour. Drain. Discard remaining sauce.

Make the dressing: In a small bowl, combine all the dressing ingredients. Mix thoroughly.

In a large bowl, toss the spinach and parsley. Transfer to 4 to 6 plates. Top with tofu and avocado. Drizzle with the dressing and garnish with the pine nuts.

Makes 4 to 6 servings

TIP

YOU CAN MARINATE THE TOFU AND MAKE THE SALAD DRESSING AHEAD OF TIME. BUT FOR THE BEST COLOR AND TASTE, CUT THE AVOCADO AND ASSEMBLE THE DISH JUST BEFORE SERVING.

Thai-Style Cabbage Salad

Napa cabbage is one of my favorite vegetables. The blanching ginseng water makes a good soup base.

4 CUPS BREWED GINSENG TEA (SEE PAGE 35)

1 SMALL NAPA CABBAGE, SHREDDED

2 TABLESPOONS CANOLA OIL

1 DRIED OR FRESH RED CHILI, SEEDED AND FINELY CUT INTO STRIPS

3 CLOVES GARLIC, MINCED

2 DRIED SHIITAKE MUSHROOMS, FINELY CUT INTO STRIPS (PAGE 27)

¼ CUP THAI SAUCE (PAGE 91)

¼ CUP ROASTED PEANUTS OR CANDIED NUTS (PAGE 102)

Place the tea in a saucepan and bring to a boil. Add the cabbage and boil for 2 minutes. Drain thoroughly. Place cabbage in a salad bowl.

Heat a nonstick cooking pan or wok over medium-high heat. Add the oil and swirl the pan to coat. Add the chili, garlic, and mushrooms and stir-fry until the mushroom strips are browned and crisp. Set aside.

Mix the sauce with the salad and toss well. Sprinkle with fried mushroom mixture and nuts.

Makes 4 to 6 servings

Pan-Fried Tofu and Orange Salad

There are so many ways you can enjoy tofu. This is a favorite of my son. The crisp, tender tofu contrasts nicely with the sweet-tart oranges.

1 (16-OUNCE) BLOCK EXTRA-FIRM TOFU

2 TABLESPOONS OLIVE OIL

½ TABLESPOON SESAME SHAKERS (SEE PAGE 58) OR WHITE SESAME SEEDS

⅛ TEASPOON SALT

2 ORANGES

4-OUNCE BAG MIXED SALAD GREENS

½ CUP CHOPPED RED ONION

½ CUP APPLE-ORANGE SAUCE (PAGE 98) OR PINEAPPLE-GINSENG SAUCE
   (PAGE 97)

Place tofu on a cutting board and press out the water. Dry with paper towels. Cut the tofu into 8 equal cubes by first cutting the block into 2 sheets, then cutting both sheets in half and then in quarters.

Heat the oil in a large frying pan. Add the sesame seeds and salt and sauté until fragrant. Add the tofu and pan-fry until golden brown, about 6 minutes. Turn the tofu and pan-fry other side until golden brown, about 3 minutes. (The second side requires less time.) Drain tofu slices on the paper towel. Cut to desired size.

Cut oranges into wedges. Use a knife to cut off the peel and cut the wedges into bite-size pieces.

Toss together the salad greens, orange pieces, and onion with Apple-Orange Sauce. Arrange the tofu slices over the salad.

Makes 6 to 8 servings

Couscous Salad with Oranges and Almonds

Couscous, a type of grain, is available in boxes and in the bulk section at supermarkets. It cooks much faster than rice. This is another salad you can serve as a meal by itself. It's good for all seasons.

1 CUP BREWED GREEN TEA (SEE PAGE 39)

½ CUP COUSCOUS

¾ CUP (½ CAN) CANNED GARBANZO BEANS,
    RINSED AND DRAINED

1 GREEN ONION (GREEN AND WHITE PARTS),
    CUT INTO 2-INCH DIAGONAL SLICES

4-OUNCE BAG SALAD MIX, SUCH AS BABY GREENS

½ CUP ORANGE AND SOY SAUCE (PAGE 89)

1 LARGE NAVEL ORANGE

¼ CUP DRIED CRANBERRIES

¼ CUP SLICED ALMONDS, TOASTED

In a 2-quart saucepan, bring the tea to a boil. Stir in the couscous. Cover saucepan and remove from heat. Let stand 5 minutes.

In a large salad bowl, mix the couscous, garbanzo beans, green onion, salad mix, and sauce. Toss to coat.

Peel and cut orange into bite-size chunks. Stir orange chunks into couscous mixture.

Garnish with cranberries and almonds.

Makes 4 servings

Spinach Salad with Oranges, Raisins, and Almonds

Spice up healthy spinach leaves with this tasty combination of sweet and tangy flavors.

½ CUP GOLDEN RAISINS

1 CUP HOT GINSENG TEA (PAGE 39)

1 LARGE ORANGE

3 TABLESPOONS OLIVE OIL

1 THICK BREAD SLICE

½ CUP SLIVERED ALMONDS

2 TABLESPOONS SUGAR

1 ¼ POUNDS BABY SPINACH LEAVES

¾ CUP ORANGE AND SOY SAUCE (PAGE 89)

¼ CUP DRIED CRANBERRIES

Place the raisins in a small bowl. Pour hot ginseng tea over them and let soak for 5 minutes. Drain.

Cut the orange into wedges, use a knife to cut off the peel, and cut the wedges into bite-size pieces.

Coat a nonstick frying pan with ½ tablespoon of the oil. Pan-fry bread on one side until golden brown. Recoat pan with another ½ tablespoon oil, pan-fry other side of bread until golden brown, 2 to 3 minutes on each side. Cut the bread into ½-inch cubes. Drain on paper towels.

In a wok or cooking pan, heat the remaining 2 tablespoons oil over medium-low heat. Add the almonds and sugar, and cook, tossing and stirring, until sugar melts and nuts turn golden brown, about 2 minutes. Be careful not to let the nut mixture burn.

Place the spinach in a salad bowl. Add the sugared nuts, sauce, and raisins. Toss and mix gently. Garnish with orange pieces, cranberries, and bread cubes.

Makes 6 servings

Melon Salad

This is a great dish for a summer gathering. If you are in a hurry, cube the melons, or use small strawberries and green grapes instead of the honeydew and watermelon. Serve this salad with grilled meat or fish.

1 CUP RIPE CANTALOUPE BALLS

1 CUP RIPE HONEYDEW MELON BALLS

1 CUP SEEDLESS WATERMELON BALLS

3 TABLESPOONS HONEY

½ CUP BREWED GREEN TEA PAGE 39)

½ TABLESPOON FRESH LEMON JUICE

3 TABLESPOONS CHOPPED MINT LEAVES

Place the melon balls in a glass fruit bowl.

Mix together the honey, tea, and lemon juice. Bring to a boil; let it cool. Spoon the sauce over the melon balls before serving. Mix gently. Garnish with mint leaves.

Makes 6 servings

TIPS

SELECTING THE PERFECTLY RIPE MELON CAN BE A DAUNTING TASK. I'VE FOUND THAT THE BEST-SMELLING MELONS TEND TO BE THE RIPEST. FIND ONES THAT SMELL LIKE THE RIPEST MELON YOU'VE TASTED. THIS METHOD WORKS FOR OTHER FRUITS TOO. SMALL, HEAVY MELONS TEND TO HAVE MORE FLESH IN PROPORTION TO THE SEEDS.

Fresh Garden Salad with Beef

To save time, replace the beef with grilled chicken breast, roasted beef, or honey ham from your deli.

1 POUND BEEF FLANK STEAK

½ CUP SPICY HONEY-BASIL SAUCE (PAGE 94)

DRESSING

3 TABLESPOONS OLIVE OIL

1 TABLESPOON DIJON MUSTARD

2 TABLESPOONS FRESH LEMON JUICE

2 CLOVES GARLIC, MINCED

1 TEASPOON GRATED FRESH GINGER

SALT AND BLACK PEPPER TO TASTE

1 MEDIUM HEAD ROMAINE LETTUCE

1 MEDIUM HEAD RED-LEAF LETTUCE

1 MEDIUM CUCUMBER, PEELED AND THINLY SLICED

1 LARGE TOMATO, SLICED

¼ CUP FRESHLY GRATED PARMESAN CHEESE

Place the beef in a shallow container. Add the sauce, cover, and marinate for 30 minutes or overnight in the refrigerator.

Make the dressing: Mix all the dressing ingredients in a salad bowl. Set aside.

Discard the marinade and grill or broil the steak to desired doneness. Transfer steak to a cutting board. Let stand 5 minutes; cut across the grain into bite-size strips.

Wash and dry the lettuce, tear into bite-size pieces, and place in a salad bowl. Add the cucumber and tomato slices.

To serve, add the dressing and toss. Divide salad among 4 salad bowls, top with the steak, and garnish with the cheese.

Makes 4 servings

Beef, Orange, and Spinach Salad

This salad is a good choice for a busy weekday night. You can put everything together in less than 10 minutes. The garlic's and ginger's yang balances the vegetables' yin.

¾ POUND LEAN ROASTED BEEF, LEFTOVERS OR FROM THE DELI

3 ORANGES, PEELED AND SEGMENTED

½ POUND FRESH YOUNG SPINACH LEAVES

¼ CUP CHOPPED FRESH CHIVES

3 CLOVES GARLIC, FINELY MINCED

1 TEASPOON MINCED FRESH GINGER

1 TABLESPOON OLIVE OIL

1 TABLESPOON GARLIC-FLAVORED RICE VINEGAR

Thinly slice the beef and set aside.

In a large salad bowl, gently mix the oranges, spinach, chives, garlic, ginger, oil, and rice vinegar.

Divide the salad among 4 to 6 serving plates. Top with the beef.

Makes 4 to 6 servings

Chickpea-Avocado Salad with Pineapple Sauce

One cup of dried chickpeas yields three cups of cooked chickpeas. If you use canned chickpeas, reduce or omit the salt. Look for canned chickpeas that are low in sodium. This simple salad makes a good light lunch.

2 CUPS COOKED OR CANNED CHICKPEAS

1 SMALL RED ONION, FINELY CHOPPED

1 SMALL RED BELL PEPPER, CUT INTO CUBES

12 BLACK OLIVES, PITTED AND CUT IN HALF

2 SMALL RIPE AVOCADOS, PEELED AND QUARTERED

½ CUP PINEAPPLE-GINSENG SAUCE (PAGE 97)

2 TABLESPOONS MINT LEAVES, CHOPPED

Rinse the chickpeas under cold water. Drain. Place in a salad bowl.

Mix in the onion, bell pepper, and olives. Arrange avocados on top. Spoon the sauce over the salad. Garnish with the mint.

Makes 4 servings

Chicken and Roasted Potato Salad

This robust salad can stand in as a main course, not just an appetizer. The leftovers are excellent for the next day's lunch, as the flavors permeate the ingredients. To save time you can also use roasted chicken from the deli or meat department. For a vegetarian version, replace chicken with flavored tofu. You will be pleased by the wonderful flavor the ginseng releases when roasting with the potatoes.

1 POUND SMALL RED POTATOES, CUT INTO 1-INCH CHUNKS,
    SKINS LEFT ON

4 TABLESPOONS OLIVE OIL

3 GINSENG TEA BAGS

SALT TO TASTE

8 OUNCES SPIRAL PASTA

1 POUND SKINLESS, BONELESS CHICKEN BREAST,
    CUT INTO 2-INCH-LONG STRIPS

¼ CUP TERIYAKI SAUCE (PAGE 90), OR PURCHASED

2 TEASPOONS CORNSTARCH

½ TABLESPOON FINELY CHOPPED FRESH GINGER

2 CLOVES GARLIC, FINELY CHOPPED

1 FRESH OR DRIED CHILI PEPPER, MINCED (OPTIONAL)

3 MEDIUM TOMATOES, EACH CUT INTO 8 WEDGES

½ CUP WATERCRESS LEAVES

½ CUP ALL-OCCASION SAUCE (PAGE 95)

Preheat the oven to 450°F (230°C). Coat the bottom of a baking dish with cooking spray. Toss potatoes with 2 tablespoons of the olive oil and contents of 1 of the ginseng tea bags. Season with salt. Roast potatoes until golden and tender, 25 to 28 minutes.

Meanwhile, in large saucepan, bring enough water to a boil to cook the pasta. Add the remaining 2 ginseng tea bags and cook pasta according to package directions. Drain and rinse under cold water.

In a bowl, thoroughly mix the chicken with teriyaki sauce and cornstarch. Heat a nonstick cooking pan or wok over medium-high heat. Add the remaining 2 tablespoons oil and swirl the pan to coat. Add the ginger, garlic, and chili and sauté until fragrant, about 1 minute. Add the chicken and stir-fry until chicken is golden brown, 2 to 3 minutes.

In a large salad bowl, toss the potatoes, pasta, chicken, tomatoes, watercress, and sauce. Serve.

Makes 8 to 10 servings

TIPS

THE RECIPE CAN BE HALVED.

THE CHICKEN BREAST IS MUCH EASIER TO CUT WHEN IT IS PARTIALLY FROZEN.

Grilled Chicken and Rice Salad

Use this as a basic recipe. Replace the grilled chicken with other grilled meat. I prefer free-range chicken.

1 POUND BONELESS, SKINLESS CHICKEN BREASTS

2 CUPS SPICY CILANTRO SAUCE (PAGE 80)

4 CUPS CURLY ENDIVE OR 1 (4-OUNCE) BAG MIXED BABY GREENS

1 CUP SNOW PEAS

1 SMALL RED ONION, THINLY SLICED

1¼ CUPS COOKED RICE

2 TABLESPOONS PINE NUTS, TOASTED (PAGE 96),
    OR CANDIED NUTS (PAGE 102)

Combine the chicken and the sauce in a bowl. Cover and refrigerate for 1 hour or overnight.

Reserve the remaining marinade. Oil the grill rack and preheat the grill to medium. Grill the chicken, turning occasionally and basting frequently with the marinade, until it is fork-tender and no longer pink throughout. Cool and slice chicken into thin strips. Set aside. Bring the remaining sauce to a boil.

Combine the endive, snow peas, and onion in a salad bowl. Add the rice. Pour the sauce over the salad and toss to mix.

Top with chicken and pine nuts.

Makes 4 servings

7. Meals in a Wok: Stir-Fried Foods

"Have you done your stir-fry?" Don't be surprised to hear two Chinese greet each other this way around mealtime. It's a friendly, nice way of asking if someone's had dinner yet. When I was growing up in China, stir-frying was a big part of my life, just as vegetables, tofu, and rice were.

As early as I can remember, I helped my grandmother arrange ingredients on a plate after she cut them. When she threw all the ingredients into the heated wok, I got my chopsticks ready. I knew that in no time I would be enjoying her delicious stir-fry.

For centuries, stir-frying has been an important cooking method among the Chinese. Fresh vegetables and rice are always the focus of the dish. Small amounts of seafood, meats, and oils are added to the dish to enhance the color and taste, keeping the meals low in fat and high in flavor.

In a couple of minutes the cold, raw food takes on a new, delicious life. The flavors you add give the dishes an infinite variety of personalities, from hot-tempered Kung Pao Chicken to enlightened Buddha's Delight.

Traditionally, preparing a stir-fry took a lot of chopping, complex seasonings, and a wok. The good news is that stir-frying is easier than ever. You can now buy precut vegetables and meats. Flavored sauces and oils lighten the burden on your spice rack. You don't even need a wok. A nonstick frying pan, a spatula, some precut foods, and a bottle of stir-fry sauce, and you are on your way.

Let your stir-fry's "personality" cater to your moods.

CHOPSTICKS

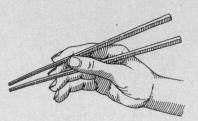

CHINESE USE CHOPSTICKS FOR MOST OF THEIR MEALS, EXCEPT WHEN EATING LARGER PIECES OF FOOD SUCH AS DRUMSTICKS OR CRABS. THEN IT'S ACCEPTABLE TO USE THE FINGERS. WHEN EATING RICE WITH CHOPSTICKS, IT IS SOCIALLY ACCEPTABLE TO BRING YOUR RICE BOWL CLOSE TO YOUR MOUTH AND SCOOP UP THE RICE WITH YOUR CHOPSTICKS. IN CHINA, DON'T ATTEMPT TO EAT YOUR RICE FROM A BOWL SITTING ON THE TABLE. YOU WILL BE THE ONLY ONE WHO IS STILL HUNGRY AT THE END OF THE MEAL.

CHOPSTICKS ARE COMMONLY MADE OF UNADORNED WOOD, BAMBOO, AND PLASTIC. SOME ARE INTRICATELY CRAFTED FROM IVORY, PORCELAIN, CLOISONNÉ, OR SILVER.

TO USE CHOPSTICKS

FOR BEGINNERS, BAND THE STICKS TOGETHER AT THE THICKER SIDE AND HOLD THEM CLOSE TO THE OTHER END. TUCK ONE STICK UNDER THE THUMB AND HOLD FIRMLY. ADD THE SECOND STICK, HOLDING IT AS YOU HOLD A PEN. HOLDING THE FIRST STICK IN PLACE, MOVE THE SECOND ONE UP AND DOWN. NOW YOU CAN PICK UP FOOD BY PINCHING IT BETWEEN THE CHOPSTICKS.

CHOPSTICK ETIQUETTE

OVER THE CENTURIES, THE CHINESE HAVE DEVELOPED SEVERAL RULES OF ETIQUETTE FOR EATING WITH CHOPSTICKS.

- THE MEAL SHOULD NOT START UNTIL THE HOST/HOSTESS OR THE OLDEST PERSON AT THE TABLE RAISES HIS CHOPSTICKS.
- CHOPSTICKS SHOULD NOT STAND UPRIGHT IN A BOWL OF RICE. THIS LOOKS TOO MUCH LIKE A TOMBSTONE ON A GRAVE.
- CHOPSTICKS SHOULD NOT BE SET LENGTHWISE ACROSS THE RICE BOWL. THIS IS CONSIDERED SYMBOLIC OF A COFFIN.
- CHOPSTICKS SHOULD NOT BE RATTLED AGAINST THE BOWL. IT'S BELIEVED THIS WILL BREAK THE WEALTH OF FUTURE GENERATIONS.
- DROPPING CHOPSTICKS WILL INEVITABLY BRING BAD LUCK; IT SYMBOLIZES DROPPING OR LOSING YOUR GOOD FORTUNE.

Techniques for Stir-frying

Stir-frying is the most common Asian cooking technique. It is also a good way to cook healthy and fast meals. With a nonstick wok or cooking pan (see page 48) you need very little oil. Most stir-fried dishes take only minutes to prepare. Because the cooking time is short, the food retains its natural flavors, nutrients, and textures.

Stir-frying can be a little intimidating at first. The following steps will ensure your successful and safe stir-frying:

- Prepare the ingredients correctly: To ensure even and fast cooking, most of these recipes call for thinly sliced or shredded ingredients. This is when you will appreciate a good set of knives. I use chopping as a form of meditation. Put on some classical music and chop, chop, chop. If you don't have time or have your own form of meditation, don't let that stop you from stir-frying. You can always use precut meats, bagged salad, and even frozen vegetables. That is what I do many weeknights.
- Assemble all the ingredients: Stir-frying is like getting on a roller coaster—once you start, there's no stopping. So make sure you have

everything cut, meats marinated, and sauces mixed. Arrange everything near the wok, including the serving plate and garnishes.

- Set the table: That's right! Stir-fried food tastes best when it's hot. You don't want your hot creation getting cold and soggy. (If dinner is delayed, place the food in a covered dish and keep it in an oven set on warm.)
- Order of cooking: Stir-frying is usually done in batches, and the order in which ingredients are added is important. Aromatic seasonings like green tea, ginger, and garlic usually go in first, followed by meats or seafood, and hard vegetables such as carrots go in before softer ones such as spinach. Add the sauce when all the food is halfway cooked.
- Begin to cook: Use high heat. Heat the wok or cooking pan for 30 seconds before adding the oil. Drizzle in the oil, usually no more than 2 tablespoons. Swirl it to coat the surface. Don't wait until the oil is too hot. If you hold your hand above the wok and can feel the heat, it's ready. If the recipe calls for dry green tea leaves, garlic, ginger, or chili pepper, this is the time to add it. With practice you can judge by the cooking sound and smell. The purpose here is to flavor the oil and release the fragrance of the seasonings.

  Quickly add the other ingredients and cover immediately to prevent splattering. Keep the food moving by giving the wok a couple of good shakes. After a couple seconds of shaking, you are safe to open the lid and start stir-frying. Most of the water has cooked off.
- Stir: Use your spatula to toss the food over the surface of the wok or pan, so that everything cooks evenly. I prefer to use one of the new heat-resistant silicone spatulas, which can resist temperatures up to 650°F (345°C).

Tasting

Don't forget to taste the dish before you put it on the serving plate. Many recipes call for salt and pepper to taste. This is the time to adjust the seasoning. I always save sesame oil for last, since its flavor tends to evaporate in high heat.

Harmony Holiday Delight

As you may know, in Chinese culture food and family are two of the most important elements of life. Food is also highly symbolic, and there's a food that symbolizes nearly every aspect of life. So of course there's a dish for family gatherings on holidays that represents the harmony among family members.

This dish, with its mix of the colorful and the savory, the spicy and the wholesome, may remind you of your own relatives. And perhaps like your own family, as the ingredients come together, they find their own harmony.

For your vegetarian guests, this delicious dish will also provide a nice holiday protein boost.

3 TABLESPOONS CANOLA OIL

5 CLOVES GARLIC, MINCED

1½ TABLESPOONS MINCED FRESH GINGER

1 FRESH RED CHILI PEPPER, MINCED

1 CUP FRESH SHIITAKE MUSHROOM CAPS,
    CUT INTO ½-INCH CUBES

2 CUPS SHELLED FRESH OR FROZEN GREEN SOYBEANS

1 CUP FROZEN WHOLE-KERNEL CORN

½ CUP SOYMILK

1 TABLESPOON RICE VINEGAR

1 CUP DRIED CHERRIES OR CRANBERRIES

SALT AND WHITE PEPPER TO TASTE

16 THIN SLICES ENGLISH CUCUMBER

16 THIN SLICES FRESH TOMATOES

2 TABLESPOONS BLACK SESAME SEEDS,
    TOASTED (SEE TIP, PAGE 200)

Heat a nonstick cooking pan or wok over medium-high heat. Add the canola oil and swirl the pan to coat. Add the garlic, ginger, chili pepper, and mushrooms. Stir-fry until fragrant, 1 to 2 minutes.

Add the soybeans. Stir-fry for 1 minute. Mix in the corn, soymilk, and vinegar and cook, stirring, until most of the liquid cooks off, 2 to 3 minutes.

Mix in the cherries. Season with salt and white pepper.

To serve: decorate the edge of a round plate with alternating cucumber and tomato slices. Top with the vegetables. Garnish with toasted sesame seeds.

Makes 8 servings

TIP

SOME SESAME SEEDS CAN BE PURCHASED ALREADY TOASTED. TO TOAST YOUR OWN SESAME SEEDS: PREHEAT THE OVEN TO 350°F (175°C). SPREAD THE SESAME SEEDS ON A BAKING SHEET IN A SINGLE LAYER. BAKE FOR 5 TO 6 MINUTES, OR UNTIL THE SESAME SEEDS ARE CRISP AND FRAGRANT.

Pan-Fried Udon Noodles with Teriyaki Sauce

Use the best green tea you can find for this dish; it will add so much flavor to the noodles. The best variety is gunpowder, so-called because the tea leaves look like little balls of black gunpowder. After you sauté the leaves they will unfurl, releasing a wonderful aroma.

9 OUNCES FRESH OR DRIED UDON NOODLES

2 TABLESPOONS CANOLA OIL

2 TEASPOONS LOOSE GREEN TEA

2 CLOVES GARLIC, FINELY CHOPPED

½ TABLESPOON MINCED FRESH GINGER

4 OUNCES BAKED, FLAVORED TOFU (PACKAGES, OR RECIPE
    ON PAGE 125), CUT INTO 1-INCH CUBES

1 MEDIUM CARROT, CUT INTO LONG MATCHSTICK-SIZE PIECES

1 MEDIUM DAIKON, CUT INTO LONG MATCHSTICK-SIZE PIECES

1 MEDIUM LEEK (WHITE PART ONLY), CUT INTO LONG
    MATCHSTICK-SIZE PIECES

3 TABLESPOONS TERIYAKI SAUCE (PAGE 90) OR PURCHASED

1 TABLESPOON RICE VINEGAR

2 TABLESPOONS SHREDDED ROASTED SEAWEED (PAGE 58) OR
    TOASTED BLACK SESAME SEEDS (PAGE 200), FOR GARNISH

Cook the noodles according to the package directions. Drain and rinse under cold water. Set aside.

Heat a nonstick cooking pan or wok over medium-high heat. Add the oil and swirl the pan to coat. Add the tea and stir-fry until fragrant, about 30 seconds. Add the garlic, ginger, and tofu. Stir-fry until tofu is golden brown, about 2 minutes. Add the carrot, daikon, and leek and stir-fry for 1 minute. Mix in the noodles, sauce, and vinegar. Cook, stirring occasionally, until noodles are heated through. Garnish with seaweed. Serve hot or cold.

Makes 4 servings

TIPS

WHEN BUYING NOODLES, CHECK THE NUTRITION LABEL AND BUY ONES THAT ARE LOW IN SODIUM. SOME CONTAIN VERY HIGH SODIUM LEVELS.

Spicy Spinach with Sesame Seeds

Both green tea and spinach are considered yin elements in Chinese cooking and medicine. This is a great dish to serve along with a red meat dish. It will help balance the yang element of the red meat. Serve hot with rice.

1½ TABLESPOONS CANOLA OIL

2 TEASPOONS LOOSE GREEN TEA

3 CLOVES GARLIC, MINCED

1 TEASPOON CHOPPED, SEEDED FRESH RED CHILI PEPPER

1 POUND FRESH BABY SPINACH

1 TABLESPOON RICE VINEGAR

SALT AND FRESHLY GROUND PEPPER TO TASTE

2 TABLESPOONS WHITE SESAME SEEDS, TOASTED
    (PAGE 200), FOR GARNISH

Add the oil to a nonstick wok or large frying pan and swirl to coat. Heat the oil over medium-high heat. Add tea and sauté until fragrant, about 30 seconds. Add garlic and pepper and stir-fry for 30 seconds.

Add the spinach; stir-fry for 2 minutes. Stir in rice vinegar and continue stir-frying until leaves are slightly wilted, about 1 minute. Season with salt and pepper. Garnish with sesame seeds.

Makes 4 to 6 servings

Wild Rice with Cranberries and Pine Nuts

I cook this dish year-round. It's a perfect side dish or stuffing for poultry or pork tenderloin. Its marriage of cranberries and pine nuts makes it a healthy alternative to ordinary bread stuffing. For your next holiday meal, give this stuffing a try.

2 CUPS WILD RICE

3 CUPS COLD SPRING WATER

2 CUPS BREWED GINSENG TEA OR GREEN TEA (PAGE 39)

4 TABLESPOONS EXTRA-VIRGIN OLIVE OIL

4 CLOVES GARLIC, MINCED

1 CUP FRESH OYSTER OR SHIITAKE MUSHROOMS, MINCED

3 MEDIUM CARROTS, CUT INTO ¼-INCH CUBES (ABOUT 2 CUPS)

½ CUP MINCED ONION

2 CELERY STALKS, CUT INTO ¼-INCH CUBES

1 CUP FRESH ORANGE JUICE

1 CUP DRIED CRANBERRIES

2 TABLESPOONS CHOPPED FRESH PARSLEY

SALT AND BLACK PEPPER TO TASTE

½ CUP PINE NUTS OR SLICED ALMONDS, TOASTED (SEE TIP, PAGE 96)

Rinse the rice thoroughly with cold water. Place the rice, water, and tea in a 6-quart saucepan. Bring rice to a boil. Reduce heat to medium-low and let it simmer, partly covered, until rice has puffed and most of liquid is absorbed, 55 to 60 minutes.

Preheat the oven to 325°F (165°C). Heat a nonstick cooking pan

or wok over medium-high heat. Add the oil and swirl the pan to coat. Add the garlic and ginseng and sauté until fragrant, about 30 seconds. Add mushrooms and stir-fry for 1 minute. Add the carrots, onion, and celery. Stir-fry until vegetables are tender, about 2 minutes.

Stir in the rice, orange juice, cranberries, and parsley. Toss to mix well.

Pour the rice mixture into a 13-by-9-inch baking dish. Cover with foil and bake until heated through and liquid evaporates, about 30 minutes. Garnish with pine nuts before serving.

Makes 11 cups

TIPS

WHILE THE RICE SIMMERS, PREPARE THE OTHER INGREDIENTS FOR THE STUFFING AND TOAST THE PINE NUTS.

THE STUFFING CAN BE MADE AHEAD. POUR THE RICE MIXTURE INTO THE BAKING PAN. COVER AND REFRIGERATE. BAKE JUST BEFORE SERVING.

Shredded Potatoes with Ginseng

This is a variation of a very popular dish from the northern part of China. In the past during the wintertime, fresh vegetables were hard to come by. Families had to live on potatoes for months. This is one of the popular ways to cook potatoes in China. I was glad to add this dish to my potato recipe collection.

1 POUND RED POTATOES, PEELED AND THINLY SHREDDED

3 TABLESPOONS CANOLA OIL

3 CLOVES GARLIC, MINCED

½ FRESH CHILI PEPPER

CONTENTS OF 2 GINSENG TEA BAGS

½ CUP FINELY CHOPPED RED ONION

2 TABLESPOONS RICE VINEGAR

SALT AND WHITE PEPPER TO TASTE

2 TABLESPOONS CHOPPED FRESH CHIVES

Soak the potatoes in cold water for 10 minutes; drain.

Heat a nonstick cooking pan or wok over medium-high heat. Add the oil and swirl the pan to coat. Add the garlic, chili pepper, and ginseng and sauté until fragrant, about 1 minute. Add the potatoes and stir-fry until potatoes are crispy, 3 to 5 minutes. Add the red onion and stir-fry until onion starts to soften, about 2 minutes. Add the vinegar and season with salt and pepper.

Garnish with the chives. Serve hot.

Makes 4 to 6 servings

Summer Tofu Delight

Tofu and tomato are a tasty combination. During the summertime in China, we ate this dish a couple of times each week. Serve with rice or noodles.

1 (16-OUNCE) BLOCK EXTRA-FIRM TOFU

2 TABLESPOONS SAVORY OIL (PAGE 81), OR CANOLA OIL

½ CUP FRESH OR DRIED SHIITAKE MUSHROOMS (PAGE 27),
   STEMS REMOVED, MINCED

¾ POUND TOMATOES, CUT INTO 1-INCH CUBES

2 TABLESPOONS SOY SAUCE

SALT AND WHITE PEPPER TO TASTE

2 GREEN ONIONS (GREEN AND WHITE PARTS), FINELY CHOPPED

Preheat the oven to 350°F (175°C). Bake the block of tofu for 30 minutes. Press out the water and cut lengthwise into 2 sheets, then cut each sheet into thirds.

Heat the oil in a wok. Add the mushrooms and tofu slices and sauté until browned. Add the tomatoes and stir-fry for 2 minutes. Add the soy sauce. Stir-fry for 1 minute. Season with salt and pepper. Garnish with the green onions.

Makes 4 servings

TIP

TWENTY PERCENT OF MODERN MEDICINES OCCUR NATURALLY IN FRUITS AND VEGETABLES. EATING FIVE SERVINGS OF FRUIT AND VEGETABLES DAILY CAN LOWER YOUR RISK OF DISEASE. A SERVING IS ABOUT ½ CUP OF COOKED OR RAW FRUIT OR VEGETABLES.

Stir-Fried Flavored Tofu and Vegetables

This is a colorful dish, accented with flavors of sesame, ginger, and cilantro. Serve with rice or noodles.

3 TABLESPOONS SAVORY OIL (PAGE 81) OR PURCHASED

4 OUNCES FLAVORED, BAKED TOFU (PACKAGED, OR RECIPE ON PAGE 125), CUT INTO 2-INCH-LONG MATCHSTICK-SIZE STRIPS

½ TABLESPOON MINCED GINGER

1 CARROT, CUT INTO 2-INCH-LONG MATCHSTICK-SIZE STRIPS

4 LARGE DRIED SHIITAKE MUSHROOMS CAPS (SEE PAGE 27), CUT INTO THIN STRIPS

1 CELERY STALK, CUT INTO 2-INCH-LONG MATCHSTICK-SIZE STRIPS

¼ CUP WATER CHESTNUTS CUT INTO 2-INCH-LONG MATCHSTICK-SIZE STRIPS

1 RED BELL PEPPER, CUT INTO 2-INCH-LONG MATCHSTICK-SIZE STRIPS

1 YELLOW BELL PEPPER, CUT INTO 2-INCH-LONG MATCHSTICK-SIZE STRIPS

2 GREEN ONIONS (GREEN AND WHITE PARTS), CUT INTO 2-INCH SECTIONS

¼ CUP SPICY HONEY-BASIL SAUCE (PAGE 94)

CILANTRO SPRIGS, FOR GARNISH

Heat a nonstick cooking pan or wok over medium-high heat. Add 1½ tablespoons of the oil and swirl the pan to coat. Spread the tofu in the pan. Reduce the temperature to medium and cook, stirring, until the tofu is lightly browned, 4 to 5 minutes. Transfer to a plate and set aside.

Increase the heat to high and heat the remaining 1½ tablespoons oil. Add the ginger and cook until fragrant, about 30 seconds. Add the carrot and stir-fry for 1 minute. Add the mushrooms, celery, water

chestnuts, bell peppers, and green onions and stir-fry for 1 minute. Stir in the tofu and sauce and heat, stirring, until vegetables are tender and crisp. Garnish with cilantro; serve hot.

Makes 4 to 6 servings

RESCUING A DISH

CHOOSE ONLY ONE OPTION IF MORE THAN ONE IS GIVEN.

TOO BLAND:

- FOR VEGETABLES—ADD A DASH OF SALT, HOT CHILI PEPPER OIL, OR CHICKEN BROTH.
- FOR MEATS—ADD A DASH OF SOY SAUCE AND VINEGAR OR MINCED GARLIC.
- FOR SEAFOOD—ADD A DASH OF FISH SAUCE, RICE WINE, OR MINCED GINGER.

TOO SALTY:

- ADD MORE FRESH OR FROZEN VEGETABLES TO THE DISH.
- ADD A DICED PEELED POTATO. IT WILL ABSORB THE EXCESS SALT.
- ADD A DASH OF VINEGAR OR SUGAR.

TOO MUCH OIL:

- ADD MORE FRESH VEGETABLES.
- DRAIN OFF THE EXCESS OIL.

TOO LITTLE OIL:

+ Use the spatula to push the food to the sides, create a hole in the center of the wok or cooking pan, and add more oil.

STICKING TO THE PAN:

+ Use the methods for too little oil.
+ Turn down the heat and add some water.

UNDERCOOKED:

+ Return food to the pan. Cook over low heat, adding more sauce or water, if needed.

OVERCOOKED:

+ Stir in some colorful, easy-to-cook vegetables such as peas, minced bell peppers, or leafy vegetables.

SAUCE TOO THICK:

+ Reduce the heat to low. Stir in a little water while the sauce is still simmering. Add water, 2 tablespoons at a time, as needed.

SAUCE TOO THIN:

+ Reduce the heat to medium-low. Dissolve 1 teaspoon cornstarch in 1 tablespoon cold water and stir into the sauce. Cook, stirring, until the sauce begins to thicken. Repeat this procedure as necessary.

NOT ATTRACTIVE:

+ Use colorful fruits and vegetables as garnishes. Be imaginative! A beautiful serving dish is always a big plus.

Spicy Corn Sauté

This is a perfect picnic and weekend dish. The leftovers can be served with rice and bread for a healthy weekday lunch.

2 TABLESPOONS CANOLA OIL

1 CLOVE GARLIC, MINCED

¼ CUP CHOPPED WHITE ONION

CONTENTS OF 1 GINSENG OR GREEN TEA BAG

2 CUPS FRESH OR FROZEN WHOLE-KERNEL CORN

1 SMALL GREEN BELL PEPPER, SEEDED AND CHOPPED

1 CUP 1-INCH LENGTHS OKRA

1 TOMATO, SEEDED AND CHOPPED

¼ CUP SOYMILK

SALT AND WHITE PEPPER TO TASTE

¼ CUP PINE NUTS, TOASTED (SEE PAGE 96)

Heat a nonstick cooking pan or wok over medium heat. Add the oil and swirl the pan to coat. Add the garlic, white onion, and ginseng and sauté until fragrant, about 1 minute.

Add the corn and bell pepper and stir-fry for 1 minute. Add the okra and stir-fry for 1 minute. Add the tomato and soymilk. Reduce heat to low and simmer, stirring occasionally, until corn is heated through and most of the sauce cooks off, about 2 minutes. Season with salt and pepper. Top with pine nuts. Serve hot.

Makes 6 to 8 servings

Buddha's Delight

This hearty meal is especially enjoyable on a cold day. Keep this recipe in mind when your vegetarian friends come for dinner.

1 (2.5-OUNCE) PACKAGE BEAN THREAD NOODLES (PAGE 55)

1 TABLESPOON CANOLA OIL

1 TEASPOON MINCED FRESH GINGER

3 CLOVES GARLIC, MINCED

CONTENTS OF 2 GINSENG TEA BAGS (OPTIONAL)

2 OUNCES OYSTER MUSHROOMS, COARSELY CHOPPED

4 OUNCES BAKED, FLAVORED TOFU (PACKAGED, OR RECIPE ON PAGE 125), CUT INTO 1-INCH CUBES

2 CUPS 1-INCH PIECES NAPA CABBAGE

½ CUP SHREDDED BAMBOO SHOOTS

½ CUP GINGER-MUSHROOM SAUCE (PAGE 85)

SALT AND WHITE PEPPER TO TASTE

2 TEASPOONS SESAME OIL

3 SPRIGS CILANTRO, CUT INTO 2-INCH PIECES

Soak the noodles in hot water until soft, about 10 minutes. Drain and set aside.

Heat a nonstick cooking pan or wok over medium-high heat. Add the oil and swirl the pan to coat. Add the ginger, garlic, ginseng, and mushrooms and sauté until fragrant, about 1 minute.

Add the tofu, cabbage, and bamboo shoots and stir-fry for 2 minutes. Add the noodles and sauce. Bring to a boil; reduce heat to medium-low, cover, and simmer. Cook until vegetables are tender, about 3 minutes. Season with salt and pepper.

Transfer to a serving bowl. Stir in the sesame oil and garnish with cilantro.

Makes 4 servings

Green Soybeans with Baked Tofu

During my childhood summers in China, early in the morning Grandmother and I sat under a shady tree and I helped her shell the fresh soybeans while listening to her fascinating stories. Now, I buy the frozen shelled soybeans in the health-food stores.

5 CUPS BREWED GREEN TEA (SEE PAGE 39)

2 CUPS SHELLED GREEN SOYBEANS

3 TABLESPOONS SAVORY OIL (PAGE 81) OR PURCHASED

1 (8-OUNCE) PACKAGE THAI OR OTHER FLAVORED BAKED TOFU (PACKAGED, OR RECIPE ON PAGE 125), CUT INTO 1-INCH CUBES

3 GREEN ONIONS (WHITE PART ONLY), CUT INTO 1-INCH LENGTHS

½ CUP MINCED RED BELL PEPPER

1 TABLESPOON SOY SAUCE

1 TEASPOON FRESH LEMON JUICE

1 TEASPOON SESAME OIL

SALT AND BLACK PEPPER TO TASTE

STEAMED RICE, TO SERVE

Place the green tea in a big pot and bring to a boil. Add the soybeans. Boil, uncovered, until bright green, about 3 minutes. Drain.

Heat a nonstick cooking pan or wok over medium-high heat. Add the oil and swirl the pan to coat. Add the tofu and stir-fry until golden-brown, about 2 minutes.

Add the soybeans and stir-fry for 1 minute. Add the green onions, bell pepper, soy sauce, lemon juice, and sesame oil. Stir-fry until heated through, 1 to 2 minutes. Season with salt and black pepper. Serve hot with rice.

Makes 4 servings

Stir-Fried Bok Choy with Shiitake Mushrooms

Many restaurants cook this dish with a base of chicken broth. Those of you who are vegetarian can enjoy a vegan version of this Cantonese delicacy.

3 DRIED SHIITAKE MUSHROOMS

2 TABLESPOONS CANOLA OIL

½ TABLESPOON LOOSE GREEN TEA

2 CLOVES GARLIC, MINCED

1 POUND BABY BOK CHOY OR REGULAR BOK CHOY,
    CUT IN HALF LENGTHWISE

½ TABLESPOON RICE WINE

2 TABLESPOONS RICE MILK OR SOYMILK

SALT AND BLACK PEPPER TO TASTE

Soak the mushrooms in warm water until they soften, about 15 minutes. Rinse the mushrooms under running water. Use your hand to squeeze out any excess water. Cut into 2-inch chunks.

Wash and drain the bok choy. Cut it lengthwise into 3-inch pieces.

Heat a nonstick cooking pan or wok over medium-high heat. Add the oil and swirl the pan to coat. Add the tea leaves and stir-fry until fragrant, about 30 seconds. Add the garlic and mushrooms and stir-fry until fragrant, about 1 minute.

Add the bok choy and cover immediately to prevent the oil from spattering. Give the pan two good shakes. Cook for 30 seconds. Remove the cover and stir-fry until bok choy leaves turn green and soften. Add rice wine and rice milk and stir-fry for 1 minute. Season with salt and pepper. Serve hot.

Makes 4 servings

ASIAN BEAUTY SECRETS

GREEN TEA

THE LATEST TREND IN TOP-OF-THE-LINE COSMETICS HAS ITS ROOTS IN VENERABLE GREEN TEA. ARE THERE OTHER EASY WAYS TO TAKE ADVANTAGE OF THOUSANDS OF YEARS OF BEAUTY WISDOM WITHOUT EMPTYING YOUR WALLET? YOU MAY WANT TO TRY THE FOLLOWING ASIAN SECRETS.

FOR YOUR HAIR AND SKIN:

- ✦ BATHE IN MINT-FLAVORED GREEN TEA FOR REJUVENATING AND COOLING THE SKIN.
- ✦ RINSE FRESHLY WASHED HAIR WITH STRONG TEA FOR SHINE AND SOFTNESS.
- ✦ USE WARM TEA TO TREAT PIMPLES, ITCHING, SWELLING, AND SKIN RASHES.
- ✦ SOAK A TOWEL IN COLD TEA; PLACE THE TOWEL ON SUNBURNED SKIN TO HELP COOL AND HEAL.
- ✦ USE STRONG BREWED TEA AS A DISINFECTANT FOR SKIN LACERATIONS.
- ✦ FOR TIRED EYES, PLACE A TOWEL SOAKED IN WARM TEA, OR BREWED TEA BAGS, ON EYES.

Spring Rice Noodles with Vegetables

Be sure to use only the freshest young vegetables for this springtime dish.

8 OUNCES DRIED RICE NOODLES (PAGE 55)

2 TABLESPOONS CANOLA OIL

3 CLOVES GARLIC, MINCED

1 TABLESPOON GRATED FRESH GINGER

4 OUNCES FLAVORED BAKED TOFU (PACKAGED, OR RECIPE ON PAGE 125),
    CUT INTO 2-INCH CUBES

8 FRESH SHIITAKE MUSHROOMS CAPS, THINLY SHREDDED

1 MEDIUM CARROT, CUT INTO 2-INCH-LONG MATCHSTICK-SIZE STRIPS

¼ CUP YOUNG GREEN BEANS, CUT INTO 2-INCH LENGTHS

½ CUP RED BELL PEPPER, CUT INTO FINE STRIPS

1 CUP FINELY SHREDDED CABBAGE

1 CUP CURRY PEANUT SAUCE (PAGE 84)

1/2 CUP BEAN SPROUTS, ENDS REMOVED

Place the noodles in a heatproof bowl, cover with boiling water, and soak for 5 minutes until soft. Drain.

Heat a nonstick chef's pan or wok over medium-high heat. Add the oil and swirl the pan to coat. Add the garlic, ginger, tofu, and mushrooms and stir-fry for 1 minute. Add the carrot, green beans, bell pepper, and cabbage and stir-fry for 2 minutes. Add the sauce, toss to coat, cover, and steam for 1 minute. Add the noodles and bean sprouts and toss together. Cover and let simmer until noodles heat through, about 1 minute. Transfer to a serving platter.

Makes 4 to 6 servings

Longevity Noodles

Use the longest noodles you can find for this recipe. The noodles represent a wish for a long and happy life. Chinese show respect toward their elders at celebrations and birthdays by serving them extra-long noodles. Remember to serve the elders first. Some of my friends don't want to admit to being "elder," so I sometimes give this honor to the person who arrived last. In this dish, ginger is in both the marinating sauce and the seasoning sauce.

8 OUNCES BONELESS, SKINLESS CHICKEN BREASTS,
   CUT INTO 2-INCH MATCHSTICK-SIZE STRIPS

½ CUP SPICY SESAME SAUCE (PAGE 78)

8 OUNCES THIN SPAGHETTI

2 TABLESPOONS CANOLA OIL

½ CUP SNOW PEAS

½ CUP THINLY SLICED CARROT

1½ CUPS CURRY PEANUT SAUCE (PAGE 84)

SALT AND BLACK PEPPER TO TASTE

2 GREEN ONIONS (WHITE AND GREEN PARTS),
   THINLY SLICED DIAGONALLY, FOR GARNISH

In a bowl, combine the chicken and Spicy Sesame Sauce. Cover and refrigerate for 30 minutes or longer.

While the chicken marinates, cook the spaghetti according to package directions. Drain and rinse with cold water to prevent sticking. Set aside.

Snap the stem ends off the snow peas and pull the stems along the top ridge to remove any fiber.

Heat a nonstick cooking pan or wok over medium-high heat. Add the oil and swirl the pan to coat. Add the chicken and stir-fry until no longer pink, about 2 minutes. Add the snow peas and carrot and stir-fry for 2 minutes. Stir in the noodles and Curry Peanut Sauce. Mix thoroughly. Season with salt and pepper. Transfer to serving dish. Garnish with green onions. Serve hot or cold.

Makes 4 servings

DO'S FOR THE KITCHEN

- Do wash vegetables before cutting.
- Do wash the cutting board with soap and hot water after cutting raw meat or seafood.
- Do dry or drain food before adding it to a heated wok or cooking pan to prevent hot oil from splattering.
- Do apply a thin coating of oil in a wok or cooking pan to add crispness, color, and flavor.
- Do read product care instructions.
- Do look in my cookbooks for ideas.
- Do enjoy cooking!

DON'TS FOR THE KITCHEN

- Don't use cooking sprays on some nonstick cookware, such as Calphalon.
- Don't place cutting knives in the dishwasher. Wash by hand and store in a wooden block.
- Don't leave raw foods uncovered and unrefrigerated.
- Don't leave cooking food unattended.
- Don't wash nonstick cookware in the dishwasher.
- Don't use metal spatulas with nonstick cookware.
- Don't hesitate to substitute ingredients in my recipes.
- Don't panic when mistakes happen. See page 209, "Rescuing a Dish."

Ginger and Orange Chicken with Fresh Vegetables

This is one of my family's favorite weeknight dinners. To cut down on the cooking time, and for more flavorful chicken, start the chicken marinating the night before. Serve over steamed rice or linguini.

1 CUP ORANGE AND SOY SAUCE (PAGE 89)

¼ CUP CORNSTARCH

1 POUND BONELESS, SKINLESS CHICKEN BREASTS,
    CUT INTO LONG, THIN STRIPS

3 TABLESPOONS CANOLA OIL

1 TABLESPOON SHREDDED FRESH GINGER

2 TABLESPOONS MINCED ORANGE PEEL (SEE TIP PAGE 220)

½ CUP FRESH SHIITAKE OR PORTOBELLO MUSHROOM CAPS,
    THINLY SHREDDED

½ CUP THINLY SHREDDED LEEK (WHITE PART ONLY)

½ CUP THINLY SHREDDED CARROT

½ CUP THINLY SHREDDED RED BELL PEPPER

SALT TO TASTE

Combine half of the sauce and the cornstarch in a medium bowl. Stir in the chicken, cover, and refrigerate for 30 minutes or overnight. Drain off extra marinade from chicken before cooking.

Arrange the remaining ingredients around the stove.

Heat a nonstick cooking pan or wok over high heat. Add the oil and swirl the pan to coat. Add the ginger and orange peel and stir-fry until fragrant, about 30 seconds. Add the chicken and stir-fry until no pink remains, 1 to 2 minutes.

Add the vegetables and stir in the remaining sauce. Reduce the heat. Stir-fry until vegetables are crisp, tender, and heated through, about 1 minute. Season with salt.

Makes 4 to 6 servings

TIP

TO PREPARE THE ORANGE PEEL, LAY THE PEEL ON A CUTTING BOARD WITH THE WHITE INNER LAYER FACING UP. WITH A SHARP PARING KNIFE, SHAVE OFF THE WHITE LAYER. MINCE THE REMAINING ORANGE PART OF THE SKIN.

Kung Pao Chicken

Serve on top of cooked pasta or steamed rice. To save time, you can buy chicken precut for stir-frying. Just make sure you ask that it be cut into thin strips. For a vegetarian version, see the variation below.

¾ POUND CHICKEN BREAST, CUT INTO MATCHSTICK-SIZE STRIPS

¾ CUP GINGER AND GARLIC SAUCE (PAGE 79)

2 TABLESPOONS CANOLA OIL

1 TABLESPOON MINCED GARLIC

1 TABLESPOON MINCED FRESH ORANGE PEEL
   (SEE TIP, PAGE 220)

4 DRIED CHILI PEPPERS

½ LARGE RED BELL PEPPER, THINLY SLICED

½ LARGE YELLOW BELL PEPPER, THINLY SLICED

1 CUP MUNG BEAN OR PEA SPROUTS, RINSED AND DRAINED

6 GREEN ONIONS (WHITE PART ONLY), THINLY SLICED LENGTHWISE

2 TABLESPOONS SOY SAUCE OR TERIYAKI SAUCE (PURCHASED, OR RECIPE ON
   PAGE 90) OR PURCHASED

3 TABLESPOONS ROASTED PEANUTS

In a bowl, toss the chicken with the Ginger and Garlic Sauce; let stand for 5 minutes. Arrange all the ingredients around the stove.

Heat a nonstick cooking pan or wok over medium-high heat. Add the oil and swirl the pan to coat. Add the garlic, orange peel, and chili peppers. Sauté until fragrant, about 1 minute.

Drain off the marinade from the chicken and discard. Add chicken to the wok. Stir-fry until browned and no longer pink in centers, 2 to 3 minutes.

Add the bell peppers and stir-fry 1 minute. Stir in the sprouts, green onions, and soy sauce. Cook, stirring frequently, until heated through, about 1 minute. Garnish with peanuts.

Makes 4 servings

VARIATION

REPLACE THE CHICKEN WITH 6 OUNCES FLAVORED BAKED TOFU (PACKAGED, OR RECIPE ON PAGE 125). YOU WON'T NEED A MARINADE SAUCE FOR THE STRONGLY FLAVORED TOFU. YOU CAN ALSO MARINATE UNFLAVORED EXTRA-FIRM TOFU IN THE MARINADE SAUCE FOR A HEALTHY VEGETARIAN DELIGHT.

Spicy Thai Noodles

This homemade famous Thai dish gives you more flavor and less fat and sodium than the restaurant creation.

9 OUNCES FRESH WIDE RICE NOODLES (PAGE 55) OR PASTA NOODLES

PASTE

2 DRIED RED CHILIES, SOAKED IN HOT WATER UNTIL SOFTENED

1 STALK LEMONGRASS (WHITE PART ONLY) CHOPPED

1 TABLESPOON CHOPPED GINGER

¼ CUP PEANUT BUTTER

½ TABLESPOON SUGAR

¼ CUP REDUCED-FAT UNSWEETENED COCONUT MILK

¼ CUP SOYMILK

1 TABLESPOON PEANUT OIL

½ POUND RAW SHRIMP, PEELED, WITH TAILS LEFT ON

4 OUNCES FLAVORED BAKED TOFU (PACKAGED, OR RECIPE ON PAGE 125),
    CUT INTO 2-INCH CUBES

1 TABLESPOON FISH SAUCE

1 CUP BEAN SPROUTS, ENDS REMOVED

2 GREEN ONIONS (GREEN AND WHITE PARTS), MINCED

2 FRESH RED CHILI PEPPERS, SEEDED AND FINELY SLICED (OPTIONAL)

3 LIMES, QUARTERED

In a big pot, cook the noodles in boiling water according to package directions. Drain and cover to keep warm.

Make the paste: Place the paste ingredients in a food processor. Process until finely chopped.

Heat the peanut oil in a small frying pan and fry the paste over low heat until fragrant, about 1 minute. Add the shrimp and tofu and stir-fry for 1 minute. Add the fish sauce and stir-fry until the shrimp turn opaque throughout and are tender.

Place the noodles in a large bowl and artistically top with shrimp mixture, bean sprouts, green onions, and chilies, if using. Top the bowl with lime quarters. Serve warm.

Makes 4 to 6 servings

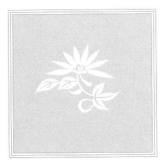

Shrimp with Candied Nuts

I first ate this dish twelve years ago when I was in San Francisco's Chinatown. Since then, I have added this one to my regular menu.

1 POUND MEDIUM RAW SHRIMP, PEELED AND DEVEINED

½ CUP SPICY SESAME SAUCE (PAGE 78)

2 TABLESPOONS CORNSTARCH

2 TABLESPOONS CANOLA OIL

1 TABLESPOON BLACK SESAME SEEDS

½ CUP CANDIED NUTS (PAGE 102)

2 TEASPOONS GRATED LEMON PEEL

In a bowl, combine the shrimp, sauce, and cornstarch and toss to coat. Cover and refrigerate for 30 minutes.

Heat a nonstick cooking pan or wok over medium-high heat. Add the oil and swirl the pan to coat. Sauté the sesame seeds until fragrant, about 30 seconds. Add the shrimp and stir-fry until shrimp turn opaque, about 2 minutes. Toss in the nuts and stir-fry for 30 seconds.

Place the shrimp mixture on a serving plate and sprinkle with the lemon zest.

Makes 4 cups

Shrimp and Curried Rice

This is a great dish for a weeknight meal. It's quick, easy, and nutritious.

2 TABLESPOONS CANOLA OIL

2 GARLIC CLOVES, MINCED

2 TEASPOONS MINCED FRESH GINGER

½ POUND PEELED LARGE SHRIMP, WITH TAILS ON

2 TEASPOONS CURRY POWDER

2 CUPS MIXED FROZEN VEGETABLES

3 CUPS COOKED RICE, USING GINSENG TEA INSTEAD OF WATER

½ CUP CURRY PEANUT SAUCE (PAGE 84)

1 TEASPOON SESAME OIL

4 SPRIGS FRESH CILANTRO, CUT INTO 1-INCH LENGTHS

Arrange the ingredients around the stove.

Heat a nonstick wok or skillet over medium-high heat. Add the oil and swirl the pan to coat. Add the garlic and ginger. Sauté until fragrant, about 1 minute. Add the shrimp and curry powder. Stir-fry until shrimp turn opaque, about 2 minutes.

Add the vegetables, rice, and sauce. Stir-fry until rice and vegetables are heated through, 4 to 5 minutes.

Stir in the sesame oil and garnish with cilantro. Serve hot.

Makes 4 servings

VARIATION
I HAVE TRIED FROZEN PEAS AND SMALL CHERRY TOMATOES INSTEAD OF THE FROZEN VEGETABLES. THE DISH LOOKED GREAT AND TASTED WONDERFUL.

Grilled Scallops with Bow Ties, Basil, and Tomato Sauce

This is a great dish for a party, an elegant dinner, or a simple weekend luncheon.

1 POUND SEA SCALLOPS, RINSED AND DRAINED

½ CUP SPICY HONEY-BASIL SAUCE (PAGE 94)

1½ POUNDS BOW-TIE PASTA

3 TABLESPOONS OLIVE OIL

½ CUP PINE NUTS

1 FRESH GREEN CHILI PEPPER, FINELY CHOPPED

4 CLOVES GARLIC, CHOPPED

½ CUP TOMATO SAUCE

2 CUPS LIGHTLY PACKED FRESH BASIL LEAVES

SALT AND WHITE PEPPER TO TASTE

2 GREEN ONIONS (GREEN AND WHITE PARTS), CHOPPED

Combine the scallops and sauce in a medium self-sealing plastic bag; seal and marinate in the refrigerator for 30 minutes or longer.

Preheat the broiler. Line a baking sheet with foil and spray with cooking spray; set aside.

In a large saucepan, cook the pasta in boiling water according to package directions. Rinse under cold water and drain well.

Meanwhile, in a nonstick wok or skillet, heat 1½ tablespoons of olive oil over medium-high heat. Add the pine nuts and sauté until golden brown, 2 to 3 minutes. Set the nuts aside in a small bowl.

Heat the remaining oil in the pan, add the chili and garlic and sauté until fragrant. Add the pasta, toss, and stir until heated through—about 2 to 3 minutes. Add the tomato sauce; toss to mix well. Stir in the basil leaves and cook, stirring, until basil leaves wilt. Season with salt and pepper.

Drain the scallops, reserving the marinade. Place scallops on prepared baking sheet. Broil until scallops brown, turning and brushing with reserved marinade once, 3 to 4 minutes on each side.

Arrange the cooked scallops on top of the pasta and sprinkle with the pine nuts and green onions. Serve hot.

Makes 4 to 6 servings

VARIATION

I OFTEN SUBSTITUTE SHRIMP OR CHICKEN FOR THE SCALLOPS, DEPENDING ON THEIR AVAILABILITY.

TIPS

IF YOU ARE HAVING A LARGE PARTY, DOUBLE OR TRIPLE THE RECIPE.

YOU CAN COOK THE PASTA AHEAD OF TIME. DRAIN AND MIX THE PASTA WITH 2 TEASPOONS OLIVE OIL TO PREVENT STICKING TOGETHER. STORE THE PASTA IN A TIGHTLY SEALED CONTAINER IN THE REFRIGERATOR.

Pan-Seared Scallops with Couscous

Couscous is a wonderful pasta frequently used in Middle Eastern cooking. Here you'll enjoy the delicate flavor of scallops combined with the spicy taste of curry paste.

2 CUPS BREWED GINSENG OR GREEN TEA (PAGE 39),
 USING 2 TEA BAGS

1 CUP COUSCOUS

¼ CUP RAISINS

2 TABLESPOONS SAVORY OIL (PAGE 81) OR PURCHASED

1 TABLESPOON CURRY PASTE

1 POUND SEA SCALLOPS

2 MEDIUM LEEKS (WHITE PART ONLY), CHOPPED

1 SMALL RED BELL PEPPER, CHOPPED

SALT AND BLACK PEPPER TO TASTE

1 GREEN ONION, CHOPPED

In a 2-quart saucepan, bring the tea to a boil. Stir in the couscous and raisins. Cover saucepan and remove from heat. Let stand 5 minutes.

In a nonstick wok or large skillet, heat 1 tablespoon of the oil and curry paste over medium-high heat until hot. Add the scallops and pan-fry until golden brown on both sides, 3 to 4 minutes.

Add the leeks and bell pepper. Stir-fry until vegetables are soft, about 2 minutes. Mix in the couscous and raisins. Season with salt and pepper. Garnish with the green onion.

Makes 6 servings

Saucy Ground Beef Wrapped in Lettuce Leaves

This dish can also be served as an appetizer or side dish. It can be made with any type of ground meat. I like to use extra-lean, naturally raised meat, which is hormone- and antibiotic-free. For a vegetarian version, substitute flavored tofu for the meat.

½ CUP MINCED LEEK (WHITE PART ONLY)

1½ TABLESPOONS MINCED FRESH GINGER

1 TABLESPOON MINCED GARLIC

CONTENTS OF 1 GINSENG TEA BAG OR ½ TABLESPOON GINSENG POWDER

1 POUND EXTRA-LEAN GROUND BEEF

25 SMALL ICEBERG LETTUCE LEAVES

2 TABLESPOONS SAVORY OIL (PAGE 81) OR CANOLA OIL

2 CUPS CANNED WATER CHESTNUTS, BLANCHED IN BOILING WATER FOR
    10 SECONDS, RINSED UNDER COLD WATER, DRAINED, AND CUT INTO
    ½-INCH CUBES

1 CUP SHELLED GREEN SOYBEANS OR GREEN PEAS

2 GREEN ONIONS (GREEN AND WHITE PARTS), CUT INTO ½-INCH PIECES

½ CUP SPICY HONEY-BASIL SAUCE (PAGE 94)

In a bowl, combine the leek, ginger, garlic, and ginseng. Add the beef and mix until the beef is combined with the other ingredients. Cover and refrigerate for 30 minutes.

Lightly flatten the lettuce leaves with the flat side of a cleaver or knife and cut into 4-inch cups. Arrange in a basket or a bowl for serving.

230   *Secrets from a Healthy Asian Kitchen*

Heat a nonstick wok or skillet over medium-high heat. Add 1 tablespoon of the oil and swirl the pan to coat. Add the beef and stir-fry, mashing and breaking it up. Cook until it changes color and separates. Transfer to a bowl.

Reheat the pan and add the remaining oil. Add the water chestnuts, soybeans, and green onions and stir-fry over high heat for about 1 minute. Add the sauce and heat through. Return the cooked beef to the pan and toss to mix with the sauce. Scoop the mixture into a serving bowl.

To serve, pass around the meat mixture and the basket of lettuce leaves; each person spoons some of the cooked meat onto a lettuce leaf, rolls it up, and enjoys.

Makes 6 servings

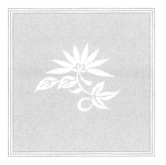

Melon and Mango with Pork

When I served this to my American friends, they were surprised. "Fruit and pork?" they asked. Yes, just as westerners serve applesauce with pork chops, Asians cook fresh fruits with meat. After sampling dishes like this in southeast China, I developed this one when I returned home.

MARINADE

2 TABLESPOONS FISH SAUCE

2 CLOVES GARLIC, MINCED

½ TABLESPOON MINCED FRESH GINGER

½ TABLESPOON FRESH LIME JUICE

1 TEASPOON CORNSTARCH

1 POUND PORK TENDERLOIN, CUT INTO LONG MATCHSTICK-SIZE STRIPS

1 CUP MATCHSTICK-SIZE STRIPS HONEYDEW MELON

1 SLIGHTLY UNDERRIPE MANGO, PEELED AND CUT INTO LONG
    MATCHSTICK-SIZE STRIPS

1 TABLESPOON FRESH LEMON JUICE

2 TABLESPOONS CANOLA OIL

3 GREEN ONIONS (WHITE PARTS ONLY), THINLY SHREDDED

SALT AND BLACK PEPPER TO TASTE

ORANGE-PEEL TWISTS

STEAMED RICE OR NOODLES, TO SERVE

Make the marinade: Mix all the marinade ingredients in a bowl. Add the pork and toss with the marinade. Cover and refrigerate for 30 minutes or longer.

In a medium bowl, toss the melon and mango strips with lemon juice. Set aside.

Arrange the remaining ingredients around the stove.

Heat the oil in a nonstick cooking pan over high heat. Add the pork (discard the marinade) and stir-fry until no pink remains, about 2 minutes.

Add the fruit and stir-fry 1 minute. Stir in the green onions. Reduce the heat and stir-fry until the ingredients are heated through. Season with salt and pepper. Garnish with orange twists. Serve over steamed rice or noodles.

Makes 4 servings

TOOTHPICKS

IN MOST ASIAN COUNTRIES, TOOTHPICKS ARE USED AS DENTAL FLOSS AS IN THE WEST. THE DIFFERENCE IS THAT IT IS ACCEPTABLE TO USE TOOTHPICKS AT THE DINNER TABLE, BETWEEN MEALS, OR RIGHT AFTER A MEAT DISH. THE POLITE WAY TO USE TOOTHPICKS IS TO COVER ONE'S MOUTH WITH ONE HAND WHILE THE TOOTHPICK IS BEING USED WITH THE OTHER.

ANOTHER MAJOR USE OF TOOTHPICKS IS FOR PICKING UP THOSE FOOD ITEMS THAT CHOPSTICKS CANNOT EASILY HANDLE, SUCH AS GRAPES OR CHOPPED FRUIT PIECES.

Pork in Green Chili Sauce

When you are pressed for time, stir-fry is one of the fastest cooking methods. Use precut and prewashed vegetables, even mixed frozen vegetables.

¾ POUND PORK TENDERLOIN, CUT INTO LONG MATCHSTICK-SIZE STRIPS

1 CUP GREEN CHILI SAUCE (PAGE 92)

1 TABLESPOON CORNSTARCH

2 TEASPOONS CANOLA OIL

1 TABLESPOON MINCED GARLIC

1 TABLESPOON MINCED FRESH ORANGE PEEL (PAGE 220)

½ LARGE RED BELL PEPPER, THINLY SLICED

½ LARGE ORANGE BELL PEPPER, THINLY SLICED

1 CUP SNOW PEAS, STRINGS REMOVED

1 CUP BEAN SPROUTS

6 GREEN ONIONS (WHITE PART ONLY), THINLY SLICED LENGTHWISE

In a bowl, toss the pork, ½ cup of the sauce, and cornstarch together; let stand for 15 minutes or longer. Drain off extra sauce from pork and discard.

Arrange the ingredients around the stove. Heat a nonstick wok or skillet over medium-high heat. Add the oil and swirl the pan to coat. Add the garlic and orange peel and sauté until garlic is golden brown, about 1 minute.

Add the pork to pan and stir-fry until brown and no longer pink in centers, 2 to 3 minutes. Add bell peppers and snow peas and stir-fry 1 minute. Stir in the remaining sauce, bean sprouts, and green onions. Stir-fry until heated through, about 1 minute. Serve hot.

Makes 4 servings

8. Outdoor Cooking: Grilled Foods

What could be better than an exotic, no-effort dinner? Even the most timid "takeout chef" can confidently barbecue a unique, delicious meal.

Like stir-frying, grilling imparts a yang influence on food. The meal becomes well balanced by serving yang food with yin sauces flavored with American ginseng (yin), green tea, vegetables, and tofu (yin), and a fruit smoothie (yin). You get delicious flavors, health benefits, and a satisfying meal all at the same time.

At my grill parties, I am frequently asked the following questions:

Is Grilled Food Healthy?

Grilled food can be healthy if we shift the focus from calorie-ridden steaks, hot dogs, and hamburgers. Tofu, fresh vegetables, fruit, mushrooms, and seafood are also good, delicious choices for grilling. At a time when data released by the Centers for Disease Control and Prevention show obesity rates continuing to increase in the United States, it is important to search for healthy alternatives.

Can Grilling Cause Cancer?

As you may know, for years researchers have been concerned about grilled food safety. Cooking meat and fish at high temperatures can produce heterocyclic amine mutagens, which may increase the risk of cancer. The good news is that adding one simple step can reduce the cancer risk: using a marinade.

Many of the distinguishing characteristics of grilled food come from the marinade used to baste the food and keep it moist and juicy when cooking. Marinating meat and fish before cooking can significantly reduce mutagen levels. According to Mark Knize, analytical chemist and principal investigator at Lawrence Livermore National Laboratory, it doesn't seem to matter how long you marinate the meat and fish. Even a brief dip in the marinade before cooking can yield this benefit. Marinated meat contained 90 percent less of the dangerous compounds than nonmarinated meat cooked the same way.

Why Is Marinating So Beneficial?

"Marinating might prevent rapid loss of water at the surface of the meat, which must occur in order for the mutagens to form," says Dr. Dashwood of the Linus Pauling Institute at Oregon State University. It doesn't seem to matter how long you marinate the meat and fish. Even a brief dip before cooking is beneficial. Nevertheless, you should still avoid overcooking meat at hot temperatures, such as those that occur when barbecuing for a prolonged time, because this is when carcinogens form.

As a bonus, all the sauces in this book contain far less fat and sodium than most commercial brands and are high in healthy components. Have fun matching the sauces (pages 78–101) with your favorite grilled foods.

General Guides to Grilling

TIPS FOR KABOBS

There are typically two types of skewers to use for kabobs: Bamboo skewers and metal skewers. Each has pros and cons. Bamboo skewers are safer and easier to handle hot off the grill than metal skewers, especially for children. Also, they are disposable. However, they must be soaked in cold water for 30 minutes before grilling to prevent them from burning. Even so, their exposed handles are still vulnerable to flame. Remember to place the uncovered handles near the cooler edges of the fire. Or, if your grill is small enough, leave the ends of the skewers outside the heated areas. If you have a larger grill and your kabob requires an extended cooking time, bamboo may not be a good choice.

Look for the flat type of metal skewers, which prevents the food from slipping as you turn them during cooking. Metal skewers are good for larger pieces of food and extended cooking times. Their longer size enables you to grill more food at the same time.

Cut foods for kabobs into uniform pieces. Group together those foods that require similar cooking times. Avoid pairing large hunks of meat or hard vegetables with quick-cooking fruits, delicate vegetables, and shellfish.

To ensure even cooking, avoid pushing foods tightly together on the skewer. Individual pieces need about ¼ inch of breathing room in order for the heat to crisp all the edges.

To remove food from the skewers, always remember to wear your oven mitts. Hold one end of the skewer with one hand and with the other hand grab the food with short-handled tongs or a potholder. Pull the food off onto serving plates.

COOKING TIPS

- Use nonstick fish holders or a nonstick tray for whole fish or fish fillets.
- Always clean the grill with a stiff wire brush before grilling.
- Before lighting the grill, spray the rack with a nonstick cooking spray, or brush it lightly with oil to prevent food from sticking to the rack.
- Marinate meats and season vegetables before grilling. If your marinade contains sugar or alcohol, use lower heat. Food will burn if the grill temperature is too high or if it is exposed to heat for too long.
- Use high temperatures for quick-cooking cuts, such as skinless, boneless chicken breasts, shrimp, and fish fillets. Use low heat for slower-cooking cuts, such as ribs and thick steaks.

- Keep the grill lid closed while grilling. It will make the grill operate more like an oven and cook the food more evenly. The food will also cook faster and use less fuel. Most important, the cover cuts off some of the oxygen, making it less likely that you will get flare-ups.
- Always wear oven mitts when handling hot food.
- Turn vegetables and fruit frequently during grilling for even cooking.
- For best results, turn fish only once during grilling

TESTS FOR DONENESS

Unlike the timing of other cooking methods, times for grilled food vary due to many factors that affect the cooking process. This includes the type of the grill and the source of the heat. How clean and airtight is your grill? What other foods are you are grilling at the same time, and how often do you peek? How windy is it in your backyard? There's also the temperature and freshness of your food, the type of marinade you are using, and individual preference for doneness to consider.

Use the cooking times in the recipes as guides, but let your nose and eyes, not the clock, help determine when the food is done to your liking. Use the following guidelines to determine doneness.

Meat: Make a small cut into the thickest part. It should no longer show pink inside. For a large cut, use an instant-read thermometer to check if the cut has reached a safe internal temperature of between 170° to 180°F (75° to 80°C) for most meats and chicken.

Fish: Test the interior of the fish with a fork; it should just begin to flake. The outside of the fish should be crispy.

Shrimp and Scallops: Shrimp and scallops should lose their translucence, becoming opaque throughout.

Vegetables and Fruit: These should be light golden brown and tender outside.

238   *Secrets from a Healthy Asian Kitchen*

Salmon Steaks with Black Sesame

Black sesame is highly regarded in Asian culture. It is used as a food, a medicine, and a beauty aid. Eating black sesame seeds in your diet, and washing your hair with a shampoo that contains black sesame, is believed to keep your hair shiny and prevent white hairs. Sesame is rich in amino acids that complement rice to make a complete protein.

½ TABLESPOON DRIED CHILI FLAKES

2 TEASPOONS LIGHT BROWN SUGAR

2 TEASPOONS GROUND CUMIN

1 TEASPOON DRIED THYME LEAVES

1 TEASPOON GARLIC SALT

2 TEASPOONS MINCED FRESH OR POWDERED GINGER

2 TEASPOONS OLIVE OIL

1 TABLESPOON FRESH LEMON JUICE

4 (¾-INCH-THICK) SALMON STEAKS (ABOUT 8 OUNCES EACH)

1 CUP BLACK SESAME SEEDS, TOASTED (SEE TIP, PAGE 200)

½ CUP MANGO-GINGER SALSA (PAGE 99)

In a small bowl, mix the chili flakes, brown sugar, cumin, thyme, garlic salt, ginger, olive oil, and lemon juice.

With a small boning knife, remove any small bones from the salmon steaks.

With your hands, rub spice mixture over both sides of the salmon steaks. Then sprinkle both sides with sesame seeds, reserving ½ cup. Oil the grill rack and preheat the grill to medium-high. Place the salmon steaks on the rack and grill, turning once, until fish flakes when tested with a fork, 8 to 10 minutes on each side. Top with remaining sesame seeds. Serve with Mango-Ginger Salsa.

Makes 4 servings

TAI CHI

THE ASIAN FOOD PYRAMID EMPHASIZES DAILY EXERCISE. (SEE PAGE 4.) AMONG THE MORE POPULAR FORMS OF EXERCISE IN CHINA IS TAI CHI. MANY CHINESE BELIEVE THAT FOR ONE TO ACHIEVE OUTER STRENGTH, ONE MUST FIRST GAIN INNER STILLNESS. TAI CHI IS THE FOUNDATION OF MARTIAL ARTS. TODAY, TAI CHI HAS SPREAD ALL OVER THE WORLD AS A FORM OF EXERCISE RATHER THAN A FORM OF FIGHTING AND DEFENSE.

EVERY DAY, MORE THAN 180 MILLION PEOPLE WORLDWIDE PRACTICE TAI CHI. SOME RESEARCHERS BELIEVE THAT PEOPLE WHO PRACTICE EVERY DAY ENJOY A LONGER, MORE ACTIVE LIFE, WITH BETTER HEALTH. OTHER EXERCISES DISSIPATE YOUR ENERGY, WHILE TAI CHI ACCUMULATES IT, LEAVING YOU FEELING REFRESHED WHEN YOU FINISH.

THE SLOW, DANCELIKE SPEED OF TAI CHI CREATES BALANCE, FLEXIBILITY, AND CALMNESS. WITH AN EMPHASIS ON DEEP BREATHING AND MENTAL IMAGERY, TAI CHI IS PRACTICED AS A SERIES OF RELAXED AND GRACEFUL MOVEMENTS PERFORMED SLOWLY BUT WITH MEDITATIVE CONCENTRATION. IT INTEGRATES YOUR MIND WITH YOUR BODY AND IS EFFECTIVE AT RELIEVING STRESS.

MORE AND MORE PEOPLE ARE BECOMING AWARE OF THE BENEFITS OF THIS BODY-STRENGTHENING AND MIND-RELAXING PRACTICE. TAI CHI HAS ALSO BEEN KNOWN TO BE A GREAT FORM OF INTERNAL EXERCISE TO HELP IMPROVE IMMUNITY AND PREVENT DISEASES.

Grilled Salmon with Spicy Honey-Basil Sauce

For a milder version, substitute Pesto Sauce (page 96).

1 CUP SPICY HONEY-BASIL SAUCE (PAGE 94)

4 SKINLESS SALMON FILLETS (ABOUT 6 OUNCES EACH)

½ CUP MINCED RED BELL PEPPER

¼ CUP CHOPPED WATERCRESS LEAVES

SALT AND WHITE PEPPER TO TASTE

1 TABLESPOON RICE VINEGAR

Spoon the sauce over the salmon, and turn to coat. Cover and refrigerate overnight or for at least 4 hours, turning twice.

Place the bell pepper and watercress in a bowl. Season with salt, pepper, and vinegar. Cover and refrigerate while the salmon cooks.

Oil the grill rack and preheat the grill to medium-high. Remove the salmon from the marinade; save the marinade.

Place the salmon on the grill rack and grill, brushing with reserved marinade occasionally, until opaque throughout, about 6 minutes on each side.

Garnish with the watercress mixture before serving.

Makes 4 servings

VARIATION

YOU CAN ALSO PLACE THE SALMON ON A SHEET OF FOIL COATED WITH COOKING SPRAY. BROIL UNDER A PREHEATED BROILER, 2 TO 3 INCHES FROM THE HEAT, FOR ABOUT 6 MINUTES ON EACH SIDE.

Almond Trout with Mango-Ginger Salsa

Living in Colorado, we get mostly frozen seafood, except for farm-raised fresh trout. During the summertime, I cook trout at least twice a week. This is one of my family's favorites.

2 FRESH TROUT (1 POUND EACH)

SALT AND FRESHLY GROUND BLACK PEPPER TO TASTE

2 GREEN ONIONS (WHITE PARTS ONLY), THINLY SHREDDED

1 TABLESPOON THINLY SHREDDED FRESH GINGER

2 TABLESPOONS CANOLA OIL

1 MEDIUM RED BELL PEPPER, CUT INTO 1-BY-4-INCH STRIPS

1 MEDIUM YELLOW BELL PEPPER, CUT INTO 1-BY-4-INCH STRIPS

¼ CUP SLIVERED ALMONDS

½ CUP MANGO-GINGER SALSA (PAGE 99)

Remove heads of the trout and scrape off the scales. Wash inside and out and pat dry with paper towels. Cut three diagonal slashes on each side of the fish. Rub fish inside and out with salt and pepper. Stuff the slashes and inside the body with the green onion and ginger.

Brush outside of fish with oil. Lightly oil the grill rack and preheat the grill to medium-high. Grill trout on both sides until browned on the outside and opaque close to the bone, 5 to 8 minutes on each side.

As the trout cook, grill bell peppers until tender and browned, 5 to 7 minutes.

Arrange grilled bell peppers around the fish. Garnish fish with almonds. Serve with Mango-Ginger Salsa.

Makes 4 servings

242   *Secrets from a Healthy Asian Kitchen*

VARIATION

THIS RECIPE WORKS WELL WHEN COOKED IN A STOVETOP GRILL PAN. ENJOY IT YEAR-ROUND.

WHICH PART OF THE FISH TO SERVE A GUEST?

FISH ARE ALWAYS SERVED AT CHINESE GATHERINGS. A WHOLE FISH SYMBOLIZES COMPLETENESS AND TOGETHERNESS. CERTAIN PARTS OF THE FISH ARE OFFERED TO THE GUEST OF HONOR. FISH HEADS AND EYES ARE OFFERED TO THE SENIOR FEMALE GUEST OF HONOR. THEY ARE VALUED DELICACIES. THE TAIL IS OFFERED TO THE MALE GUEST OF HONOR. IT IS CONSIDERED TO BE THE MOST ACTIVE PART OF THE FISH AND SYMBOLIZES ENERGY AND POWER. THE HEAD AND TAIL CONTAIN SOME OF THE JUICIEST AND MOST FLAVORFUL BITS OF MEAT. IF YOU CHOOSE NOT TO ACCEPT HONORABLE GUEST DUTY, IT IS ALWAYS SAFE AND PERMISSIBLE TO DELEGATE THE HONOR TO THE OLDEST PERSON AT THE TABLE.

Crispy Stuffed Whole Trout

Are you always impressed when cooks bring to the table a whole fish? Now you can serve it that way too. Grilling the fish instead of pan-frying it will save you cleaning time in the kitchen and cut down on the fat. You can also broil the fish in your oven.

2 WHOLE TROUT ($\frac{3}{4}$ POUND EACH), CLEANED AND SCALED, WITHOUT HEADS

SALT AND BLACK PEPPER TO TASTE

3 TABLESPOONS FINELY SHREDDED FRESH GINGER

3 GREEN ONIONS (GREEN AND WHITE PARTS), FINELY SHREDDED

3 SPRIGS CILANTRO, CUT INTO 2-INCH-LONG PIECES

1 TABLESPOON LOOSE GREEN TEA, SOAKED IN BOILING WATER AND DRAINED

1½ FRESH RED CHILI PEPPERS, FINELY SHREDDED

2 TABLESPOONS CANOLA OIL

1 SMALL YELLOW BELL PEPPER, CUT INTO 2-INCH CUBES

1 SMALL RED BELL PEPPER, CUT INTO 2-INCH CUBES

½ CUP THAI SAUCE (PAGE 91)

Cut three or four quarter-inch-deep diagonal slashes along both sides of each fish. Dry the outside of each fish with a paper towel.

Rub salt and pepper into the slashes and inside the body cavity of each fish. Stuff half of the ginger, green onions, cilantro, tea leaves, and chili into each slash and inside the body cavity of each fish.

Oil the grill rack and preheat the grill to medium-high. Place both fish on the rack and partly cover. Grill the fish until the skin is crispy brown, 5 to 8 minutes. Turn fish and place the bell peppers around

244   *Secrets from a Healthy Asian Kitchen*

them. Grill the other sides until the fish are brown and crisp, and the peppers are browned. Transfer the fish to a serving plate and arrange the peppers around or on top of the fish.

Meanwhile, heat the sauce in a small saucepan. Bring to a boil. Pour sauce over the fish and bell peppers. Serve hot.

Makes 4 servings

VARIATION

TO BROIL THE FISH, PREHEAT THE BROILER. BRUSH EACH SIDE OF THE FISH WITH CANOLA OIL. SET THE FISH IN A NONSTICK BAKING DISH THAT HAS BEEN LIGHTLY COATED WITH COOKING SPRAY. BROIL THE FISH ON THE MIDDLE RACK UNTIL THE SKIN CRISPS AND BROWNS, 10 TO 13 MINUTES ON EACH SIDE.

Sea Bass in Wine Sauce with Bananas

If you can't find fresh sea bass fillets, use any white fish fillets. A nonstick grill tray is a very useful tool to have. Use it for small vegetables and delicate fish fillets.

4 SEA BASS FILLETS (6 OUNCES EACH)

1 CUP WHITE WINE SAUCE (PAGE 87)

2 LARGE BANANAS

1½ TABLESPOONS BUTTER, MELTED

1 CUP MANGO-GINGER SALSA (PAGE 99)

In a large bowl, marinate the fish in the wine sauce in the refrigerator for 1 hour.

Oil a nonstick grill tray and place on the rack of a grill heated to medium-low. Grill until fish flakes when tested with a fork, 6 to 8 minutes on each side.

Wrap the banana in foil and grill alongside the fish until soft, about 8 minutes. Cut into big chunks, peeled.

Place the fish and bananas chunks on a serving plate. Drizzle melted butter on banana and garnish fish with Mango-Ginger Salsa.

Makes 4 servings

Apple-Orange-Glazed Shrimp Kabobs

These kabobs go well with salad and pasta dishes. End your meal with a cold drink from the dessert section. It will leave you feeling fresh and cool.

1 ½ POUNDS FRESH OR FROZEN LARGE SHRIMP

4 MEDIUM ORANGES, UNPEELED, CUT INTO CHUNKS

12 CHERRY TOMATOES

4 GREEN ONIONS (GREEN AND WHITE PARTS),
    CUT INTO 1 ½-INCH LENGTHS

1 CUP APPLE-ORANGE SAUCE (PAGE 98)

1 TABLESPOON CHIVES, MINCED, FOR GARNISH

Thaw shrimp, if frozen. Peel shrimp, leaving tails on, and devein. Wash and pat dry with paper towels.

Alternately thread shrimp, oranges, tomatoes, and green onions onto 6 (12-inch-long) skewers; brush with sauce. (See page 236 for kabob tips.)

Oil the grill rack and preheat the grill to medium. Place the kabobs on the rack and grill, turning and basting with remaining sauce, until shrimp turn opaque, 5 to 7 minutes on each side. Turn and brush often with sauce.

Arrange the skewers on a platter. Garnish with the chives. Heat the remaining sauce to a boil and serve as a dipping sauce.

Makes 6 kabobs

VARIATION

YOU CAN ALSO PLACE THE SKEWERS ON A SHEET OF FOIL COATED WITH COOKING SPRAY. BROIL UNDER A PREHEATED BROILER, 2 TO 3 INCHES FROM THE HEAT, FOR ABOUT 7 MINUTES ON EACH SIDE.

TIPS: ALL ABOUT SHRIMP

THE CHINESE LOVE SHRIMP. IT IS VIEWED AS HAVING A COOLING EFFECT (YIN).

YOU CAN BUY SHRIMP COOKED OR UNCOOKED; PEELED OR UNPEELED; UNPEELED WITH OR WITHOUT TAILS; LARGE, MEDIUM, OR SMALL. DON'T FEEL OVERWHELMED. THE RULE OF THUMB IS THAT THE LARGER THE SIZE OF THE SHRIMP, THE MORE MONEY YOU PAY. UNPEELED AND UNCOOKED SHRIMP ARE MORE FLAVORFUL BUT TAKE MORE PREPARATION TIME. THE COOKED AND PEELED SHRIMP ARE LESS TASTY BUT ARE IDEAL FOR A BUSY COOK'S LAST-MINUTE MEAL.

IN GENERAL, I USE A LOT OF PEELED UNCOOKED SHRIMP FOR WEEKNIGHT COOKING TO SAVE TIME, AND UNPEELED FOR WEEKEND MEALS. I DON'T LIKE TO USE PRECOOKED SHRIMP.

BECAUSE FRESH SHRIMP DETERIORATES IN A COUPLE OF DAYS, 98 PERCENT OF THE SHRIMP SOLD ON THE MARKET HAS BEEN FROZEN. LOOK FOR SHRIMP THAT ARE FIRM AND FREE OF ODOR.

Grilled Orange-Ginger Shrimp

I serve this dish all year round. You can easily cook it under a broiler in your oven or use a stovetop grill.

MARINADE

½ CUP FRESH ORANGE JUICE

2 TEASPOONS GRATED ORANGE PEEL

2 TABLESPOONS SEASONED RICE VINEGAR

2 TABLESPOONS SOY SAUCE

1 TABLESPOON CANOLA OIL

1 TABLESPOON MINCED FRESH GINGER

1 GREEN ONION, MINCED

2 TEASPOONS CHOPPED FRESH CILANTRO LEAVES

1 FRESH RED CHILI PEPPER, MINCED

1 POUND LARGE RAW SHRIMP, PEELED AND DEVEINED

4 LARGE ORANGES, PEELED, CUT INTO CHUNKS

STEAMED RICE OR NOODLES

Make the marinade: Combine the marinade ingredients in a bowl. Add the shrimp and toss to coat. Cover and refrigerate for 30 minutes.

Remove the shrimp from the marinade, reserving marinade.

Oil a nonstick grill tray and place on the rack of a grill heated to medium-low. Add the shrimp to the grill tray and grill, turning and basting with remaining marinade, until shrimp turn opaque, 5 to 7 minutes on each side. Add the orange chunks and toss to combine. Grill just until oranges are warmed. Serve with rice or noodles.

Makes 6 servings

VARIATION

YOU CAN ALSO PLACE THE SHRIMP ON A SHEET OF FOIL COATED WITH COOKING SPRAY. BROIL UNDER A PREHEATED BROILER, 2 TO 3 INCHES FROM THE HEAT, ABOUT 3 MINUTES ON EACH SIDE UNTIL SHRIMP TURN OPAQUE.

Grilled Shrimp with Roasted Pepper–Green Tea Sauce

This is one of my favorite dishes. The green tea helps to bring out the best flavor of the shrimp. Use the freshest shrimp you can obtain.

1 POUND FRESH LARGE SHRIMP

2 TABLESPOONS CANOLA OIL

1 ½ TABLESPOONS LOOSE GREEN TEA

1 TABLESPOON MINCED FRESH GINGER OR
    ½ TABLESPOON GINGER POWDER

1 TABLESPOON MINCED GARLIC

2 TABLESPOONS RICE WINE

1 TABLESPOON FISH SAUCE

½ CUP ROASTED PEPPER–GREEN TEA SAUCE (PAGE 101)

Peel shrimp, leaving tails on, and devein. Wash and pat dry with paper towels.

In a bowl, mix the shrimp, green tea, ginger, garlic, rice wine, and fish sauce. Cover and refrigerate for 1 hour.

Preheat the grill to medium. Oil a nonstick grill tray and place on the grill rack. Grill, turning and brushing often with sauce, until the shrimp turn opaque, about 3 minutes on each side. Serve with the sauce.

Makes 4 servings

VARIATION

YOU CAN ALSO PLACE THE SHRIMP ON A SHEET OF FOIL COATED WITH COOKING SPRAY. BROIL UNDER A PREHEATED BROILER, 2 TO 3 INCHES FROM THE HEAT, FOR 2 TO 3 MINUTES ON EACH SIDE.

Scallop Kabobs with Onion and Peppers

For a well-balanced meal, serve this dish with rice, noodles, or grilled tortillas.

1 POUND FRESH OR FROZEN SEA SCALLOPS

1 CUP SPICY HONEY-BASIL SAUCE (PAGE 94)

1 LARGE RED ONION, CUT INTO CHUNKS

1 MEDIUM YELLOW BELL PEPPER, CUT INTO CHUNKS

1 MEDIUM GREEN PEPPER, CUT INTO CHUNKS

1 TABLESPOON MINCED WATERCRESS

Thaw scallops, if frozen. Wash and pat dry with paper towels.

Place ½ cup of the sauce and the scallops in a container. Toss to coat. Cover and marinade in the refrigerator for 1 to 2 hours.

Drain the scallops, reserving the marinade. Alternately thread scallops, onion, and peppers onto 6 (12-inch-long) skewers; brush with sauce. (See Tips for Kabobs, page 236.)

Oil the grill rack and preheat the grill to medium. Place the kabobs on the rack and grill, turning and basting with remaining marinade, until scallops turn opaque, 3 to 4 minutes on each side.

Garnish with watercress. Heat remaining ½ cup sauce to a boil and use for dipping.

Makes 4 servings

VARIATION

YOU CAN ALSO PLACE THE KABOBS ON A SHEET OF FOIL COATED WITH COOKING SPRAY. BROIL UNDER A PREHEATED BROILER, 2 TO 3 INCHES FROM THE HEAT, FOR 3 TO 4 MINUTES ON EACH SIDE.

TIPS: HOW TO CHOOSE SCALLOPS

THERE ARE THREE BASIC TYPES OF SCALLOPS: FRESH SEA, FRESH BAY, AND DRIED SEA OR BAY. SEA SCALLOPS ARE LARGER AND GOOD FOR GRILLING OR PAN-FRYING. BAY SCALLOPS ARE SMALLER AND MORE DELICATE. THEY ARE GOOD FOR SOUPS, STEWS, AND STIR-FRIED FOODS. LIKE SHRIMP, THE LARGER THE SCALLOP SIZE THE MORE EXPENSIVE.

LOOK FOR FRESH SCALLOPS THAT ARE FIRM AND FREE OF FISHY OR SOUR SMELLS. IF YOU CAN'T FIND GOOD FRESH SCALLOPS, QUICK-FROZEN ONES ARE ALWAYS ANOTHER GOOD CHOICE.

CHINESE COOKING USES DRIED SCALLOPS. YOU CAN BUY THEM AT ASIAN STORES. THEY LOOK LIKE FRESH SCALLOPS, EXCEPT FOR THEIR GOLDEN, SHINY COLOR. THEY ARE MUCH MORE EXPENSIVE THAN THE FRESH ONES, BUT MORE FLAVORFUL. USE THEM IN SOUPS AND STEWS AND TO FLAVOR DISHES.

Grilled Marinated Shiitake Mushrooms

With growing scientific data demonstrating mushrooms' health benefits, now you can easily buy fresh shiitake mushrooms in health-food stores and in Asian sections of regular grocery stores. Try to get the largest mushrooms for this dish. If you can't find shiitake, use portobello mushrooms. Serve this as a side dish or sandwich filling along with grilled or fresh vegetables and sliced cheese.

1 POUND LARGE FRESH SHIITAKE MUSHROOMS

MARINADE

½ CUP EXTRA-VIRGIN OLIVE OIL

SALT AND FRESHLY GROUND PEPPER TO TASTE

2 CLOVES GARLIC, MINCED

2 GREEN ONIONS (WHITE PART ONLY), MINCED

Wash and drain mushrooms. Place in a bowl.

Make the marinade: Combine all ingredients and add the marinade to the mushrooms. Cover and refrigerate for 4 hours.

Oil the grill rack and preheat the grill to medium-low. Grill the mushrooms caps, brushing with marinade occasionally, until lightly browned on both sides, about 5 minutes on each side.

Makes 4 servings

Grilled Zucchini with Tomatoes

This dish goes well with grilled meat or served as a side dish with bread and pasta.

1 MEDIUM GREEN ZUCCHINI

1 YELLOW ZUCCHINI

½ POUND CHERRY TOMATOES

3 TABLESPOONS OLIVE OIL

3 CLOVES GARLIC, MINCED

CONTENTS OF 3 GINSENG TEA BAGS

1 TABLESPOON RED VINEGAR

1 FRESH RED CHILI PEPPER, CHOPPED

SALT AND WHITE PEPPER TO TASTE

Wash and dry zucchini and tomatoes. Bias-cut the zucchini into 1-inch-thick slices.

Place the zucchini, tomatoes, and remaining ingredients in a bowl; toss to coat. Cover and marinate in the refrigerator for 2 hours.

Oil a nonstick vegetable grilling tray and preheat the grill to medium. Place the vegetable mixture in the grilling tray. Grill the vegetables, turning occasionally, until golden and tender, 4 to 6 minutes.

Makes 6 servings

Grape Leaf–Wrapped Tofu in Thai Sauce

During my childhood in China, we didn't have a refrigerator. In wintertime Grandmother always placed a couple blocks of tofu outdoors on the windowsill. The next day we would have a meal made with frozen tofu.

Today I have one section of my freezer devoted to frozen tofu. It will last several months. As the tofu freezes, its color and texture alter. The color changes from white to tan. It will have a firmer, spongier, chewier texture—more similar to lean, tender meat than to unfrozen tofu. It is also easier to squeeze out the water and less delicate to handle. Best of all, it brings back my childhood memories.

1 (16-OUNCE) BLOCK EXTRA-FIRM TOFU

1 CUP THAI SAUCE (PAGE 91)

16 FRESH LARGE GRAPE LEAVES (PAGE 53)

1 LEMONGRASS STALK, BOTTOM 6 INCHES ONLY, MINCED

2 TABLESPOONS AMERICAN GINSENG, MINCED,
   OR CONTENTS OF 2 GINSENG TEA BAGS

Place the tofu in its package in the freezer overnight. Let it thaw in a refrigerator or in a bowl of cold water. Drain tofu from the packaged water. Rinse under cold water.

Place tofu on a cutting board and press out excess water. Cut tofu into 4-inch cubes.

In a container, toss tofu with the sauce to coat. Cover and marinate in the refrigerator for 3 hours. Turn once.

In a large pot, bring 6 cups of water to a boil. Add grape leaves and boil until leaves soften and turn bright green, 1 to 2 minutes.

Drip-dry grape leaves. Place grape leaves on an 8-inch-square piece of foil, slightly overlapping 2 leaves, place one piece of tofu in the middle and garnish with some lemongrass and ginseng. Tightly fold over the leaf's four corners. Repeat with remaining ingredients. Oil the grill racks and preheat grill to medium. Place grape leaves on the rack and grill until tofu is heated through, about 8 minutes on each side. Serve hot.

Makes 4 to 6 servings

VARIATION

ALTERNATIVELY, YOU CAN COOK THIS DISH IN A STOVETOP GRILL PAN. OIL THE GRILL PAN AND GRILL THE FILLED GRAPE LEAVES ON EACH SIDE UNTIL TOFU COOKS THROUGH. IF YOU DON'T HAVE GRAPE LEAVES, USE FOIL INSTEAD.

Tofu and Vegetable Kabobs with Curry Peanut Sauce

If you go to Indonesia, most likely you will find street vendors selling strips of marinated tofu, meat, seafood, vegetables, and fruit on skewers. Usually, they are served with a peanut sauce. I like the tofu the most, since it captures the exotic taste of the sauce.

1 (1-POUND) BLOCK EXTRA-FIRM TOFU, DRAINED

1½ CUPS CURRY PEANUT SAUCE (PAGE 84)
   OR SPICY CILANTRO SAUCE (PAGE 80)

1 RED BELL PEPPER, CUT INTO 1-INCH SQUARES

1 GREEN BELL PEPPER, CUT INTO 1-INCH SQUARES

2 WHITE ONIONS, CUT INTO 1-INCH CUBES

Preheat the oven to 400°F (205°C). Bake the tofu on an oiled ovenproof dish for 30 minutes. Slice the tofu in half. Cut each half in quarters lengthwise, then cut crosswise, into ¾-inch cubes.

In a large bowl, combine the tofu, sauce, bell peppers, and onion. Cover and marinate in the refrigerator for 2 hours, turning gently twice. Soak 8 (10-inch) bamboo skewers in water for at least 30 minutes.

Thread alternating pieces of tofu, peppers, and onion on the skewers. Preheat a stovetop or outdoor grill to medium. Place the kabobs on the grill and cook until the kabobs are brown and crisp, 3 to 4 minutes on each side.

Makes 4 servings

VARIATION

YOU CAN ALSO PLACE THE KABOBS ON A SHEET OF FOIL COATED WITH COOKING SPRAY. BROIL UNDER A PREHEATED BROILER, 2 TO 3 INCHES FROM THE HEAT, FOR 2 TO 3 MINUTES ON EACH SIDE.

TIP

BAKING THE TOFU HELPS STABILIZE IT. USE REGULAR TOFU. SILKEN TOFU WILL BE TOO FRAGILE.

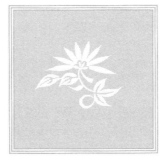

Beef and Vegetable Kabobs

There are many flavored green teas available today. Choose flavors that fit your taste. I like lemon-flavored green tea for this dish. You can also use decaffeinated green tea. Research has shown that decaffeinated green tea delivers all the health benefits of regular green tea. For a seafood or vegetarian version, replace the beef with 1 pound of sea scallops, shrimp, or tofu.

1 POUND BEEF TENDERLOIN

1 FRESH RED CHILI PEPPER, MINCED

1 TABLESPOON FINELY MINCED LEMONGRASS (WHITE PART ONLY)

3 CLOVES GARLIC, MINCED (ABOUT 1 TABLESPOON)

CONTENTS OF 2 GREEN TEA BAGS

2 TABLESPOONS LOW-SODIUM SOY SAUCE

1 TABLESPOON HOT-PEPPER SESAME OIL

1 TABLESPOON FRESH LEMON JUICE

1 MEDIUM WHITE ONION, CUT INTO 1-INCH CHUNKS

1 MEDIUM YELLOW SQUASH, CUT INTO 1-INCH CHUNKS

½ POUND CHERRY TOMATOES

1 CUP ROASTED PEPPER–SUN-DRIED TOMATOES SAUCE (PAGE 100)

COOKED NOODLES OR RICE

Cut beef into 1-inch cubes. Place the cubes of beef in a bowl. Add the chili, lemongrass, garlic, tea, soy sauce, oil, and lemon juice. Toss to coat. Cover and refrigerate for 3 to 4 hours or overnight. If using wooden skewers, presoak them in cold water for 30 minutes.

Alternately thread the beef, onion, squash, and tomatoes onto skewers.

Oil the grill rack and preheat the grill to medium-low. Add the

kabobs to the rack and grill on both sides until the beef is no longer pink and the vegetables are tender and lightly browned, 6 to 7 minutes on each side. Serve with the sauce and noodles or rice.

Makes 8 kabobs

TIP

YOU CAN ALSO COOK THIS DISH IN YOUR OVEN. JUST SET THE OVEN TO BROIL AND SET THE SKEWERS ON THE MIDDLE RACK, ON A SHEET OF FOIL THAT HAS BEEN COATED WITH CANOLA OIL SPRAY.

Steaks with Spicy Sesame Sauce

After you taste these steaks, you may never want to eat steak any other way. You can also chop up the cooked steaks, mix them with the sautéed topping, and serve over a salad.

4 LEAN BEEF FILLET STEAKS (4 OUNCES EACH)

⅓ CUP SPICY SESAME SAUCE (PAGE 78)

TOPPING

2 TEASPOONS CANOLA OIL

3 TABLESPOONS CHOPPED FRESH GINGER

4 GREEN ONIONS (GREEN AND WHITE PARTS), CHOPPED

½ CUP FRESH MUSHROOMS, CHOPPED

2 FRESH RED CHILI PEPPERS, SEEDED AND MINCED

SALT AND BLACK PEPPER TO TASTE

Trim any fat from the steaks and place in a shallow container. Add the sauce to the steaks, cover, and marinate in the refrigerator for 30 minutes.

Oil the grill rack and preheat the grill to high. Grill steaks on both sides, brushing with marinade occasionally, 6 minutes on each side for medium-rare, or until desired doneness.

Meanwhile, make the topping: Mix all the ingredients in a bowl. Preheat a nonstick grill pan over medium-high heat, add the topping mixture, and grill until vegetables are soft and fragrant, about 2 minutes.

Garnish steaks with topping and serve.

Makes 4 servings

Barbecued Sesame Ribs

Every time I cook this dish, I have to double the recipe. Otherwise when I bring it to the table my son claims he is in charge of how many ribs the rest of us should get. He likes to keep most of them for himself.

2 POUNDS BABY BACK RIBS

2 CUPS TERIYAKI SAUCE (PAGE 90)
OR APPLE-ORANGE SAUCE (PAGE 98)

2 TABLESPOONS WHITE SESAME SEEDS,
TOASTED (SEE TIP, PAGE 200)

Wash the ribs, pat dry with paper towels, and cut them into individual pieces. Mix the ribs and sauce in a large container. Cover and marinate in the refrigerator overnight or for at least 4 hours.

Remove the ribs from marinade. Save the sauce for basting.

Oil the grill rack and preheat the grill to medium-low. Place the ribs on the rack and grill, basting with remaining marinade, until the ribs are golden brown, tender, and no longer pink inside, 12 to 15 minutes on each side. Baste frequently with the sauce while grilling. Sprinkle with the sesame seeds and serve while hot.

Makes 4 servings

Grilled Skewered Beef in Pineapple-Ginseng Sauce

Serve this dish with salad, or on top of noodles or rice, or wrapped inside lettuce leaves. It makes a good summer picnic and workday lunch.

1 POUND BONELESS BEEF SIRLOIN STEAK

1 FRESH RED CHILI PEPPER, MINCED

4 STALKS LEMONGRASS, WHITE PART ONLY, FINELY CHOPPED

3 CLOVES GARLIC, MINCED

CONTENTS OF 2 GINSENG TEA BAGS

2 TABLESPOONS OLIVE OIL

SALT TO TASTE

¾ CUP PINEAPPLE-GINSENG SAUCE (PAGE 97)

Cut the steak into long thin strips about 1 inch wide. Place the steak in a bowl. Add the chili pepper, lemongrass, garlic, ginseng, oil, and salt. Mix well. Cover and refrigerate for 3 to 4 hours or longer.

Presoak about 8 bamboo skewers in cold water for 30 minutes.

Thread the steak strips on the skewers, passing the skewer through the steak several times.

Oil the grill rack and preheat the grill to medium-low. Brush the kabobs with the Pineapple-Ginseng Sauce and place on the grill rack. Grill the skewered beef on both sides, brushing with sauce again before turning, until browned, 5 to 6 minutes on each side. Heat the remaining sauce and serve with the kabobs.

Makes 4 servings

VARIATION

ALTERNATIVELY, YOU CAN COOK THIS DISH IN YOUR OVEN. PREHEAT THE BROILER AND PLACE THE SKEWERED BEEF ON THE MIDDLE RACK ON A SHEET OF FOIL THAT HAS BEEN SPRAYED WITH COOKING SPRAY.

Barbecued Ginseng Chicken Breasts

While you grill the chicken, the ginseng releases a wonderful aroma and gives the chicken a delicious flavor. Serve with pasta, grilled vegetables, or a salad.

4 MEDIUM BONELESS, SKINLESS CHICKEN BREASTS

1 ½ CUPS SPICY HONEY-BASIL SAUCE (PAGE 94)

CONTENTS OF 4 AMERICAN GINSENG TEA BAGS

Wash the chicken and pat dry with paper towels. Cut a couple of inch-long slashes on the chicken; this lets the marinade penetrate. Place chicken in a large container. Pour ½ cup of the sauce over the chicken. Toss to coat. Cover and let chicken marinate in the refrigerator for at least 4 hours or overnight.

Place the ginseng in a shallow bowl.

Remove the chicken from the marinade and dip it in the ginseng, coating it. Oil the grill rack and preheat the grill to medium-low. Place the chicken on the rack and grill until cooked through and no longer pink, 15 to 20 minutes on each side. Turn once halfway through.

In a small saucepan, bring the remaining sauce to a boil; serve over the chicken.

Makes 4 servings

TIP

TO MARINATE THE CHICKEN AS LONG AS OVERNIGHT, IT HAS TO BE VERY FRESH. STORE THE MARINATING CHICKEN IN THE COLDEST PART OF THE REFRIGERATOR, TYPICALLY THE MEAT COMPARTMENT.

Grilled Chicken with Ginger-Mushroom Sauce

The flavor is best if you can marinate the chicken overnight. When shredded, the grilled chicken also makes a good topping for wrappers and salads.

4 MEDIUM BONELESS, SKINLESS CHICKEN BREAST HALVES

1½ CUPS GINGER-MUSHROOM SAUCE (PAGE 85)

GRILLED VEGETABLES OR PASTA, TO SERVE

Toss the chicken with 1 cup of the sauce, cover, and refrigerate for at least 2 hours or overnight.

Remove the chicken from the marinade.

Oil the grill rack and preheat the grill to medium. Grill chicken, turning and brushing with the remaining marinade halfway through grilling, until chicken is fork-tender and loses its pink color throughout, about 8 to 10 minutes each side.

Let chicken cool, and cut into strips. In a small saucepan, bring remaining ½ cup sauce to a boil. Serve chicken with sauce and grilled vegetables as a filling for wrappers, or with pasta.

Makes 4 servings

9. Sweet Temptations

Did you know that tea is the Chinese beverage of choice for accompanying meals? Or that desserts aren't just served at the end of meals? They are commonly served as an afternoon snack with tea, or for special occasions throughout the day.

If you are familiar with Asian cuisine, you already know that Asian desserts are very different from western desserts. They are lighter and less sugary. The central ingredients are fresh fruit and sweet rice. Asian desserts emphasize the natural sweetness of the ingredients rather than overwhelming them with refined sugars. In general, desserts provide a little yin at the end of a meal to calm the digestive system and refresh the mouth after the main dishes.

Asian desserts are eaten in moderation. Too many sweets between meals dull your appetite. Afternoon snacks are always served with tea. Enjoy small bites between sips, to fully appreciate the delicacy of the sweet alongside the unique flavor of the tea.

Homemade ice creams and fruit smoothies are an ideal way to satisfy your craving for a sweet treat that won't pile on that extra weight. Always use the freshest fruit you can find.

In this chapter I'll share with you some of my favorite desserts and drinks. The best part is that you won't feel guilty after you indulge yourself, because these simple and elegant desserts are so good for you.

Rice Pudding with Almond and Coconut

There are many variations of rice pudding. This simple, luscious one is my favorite. If you are in a hurry, use leftover or instant rice.

1 CUP WHITE RICE

2 TEASPOONS MINCED FRESH GINGER

6 CUPS SOYMILK

2 CUPS REDUCED-FAT, UNSWEETENED COCONUT MILK (PAGE 52)

½ TEASPOON GROUND CINNAMON

HONEY TO TASTE

⅓ CUP SLICED ALMONDS, TOASTED

½ CUP GOLDEN RAISINS

Rinse the rice thoroughly with cold water.

Put the rice, ginger, and soymilk in a large heavy pot. Bring to a boil. Reduce the heat to low; partially cover the pan. Simmer, stirring occasionally, for 40 minutes.

Stir in the coconut milk, cinnamon, and honey. Simmer until the pudding turns into thick porridge, about 10 minutes.

Top with almonds and raisins. Serve warm or cold.

Makes 6 to 8 servings

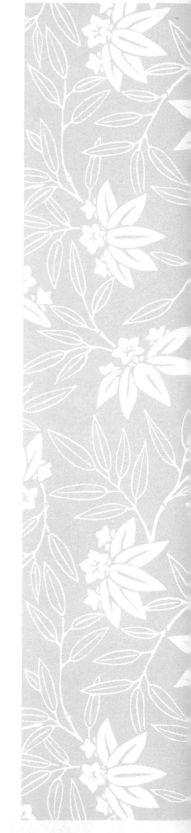

Sweet Eight-Treasure Rice Pudding

This is a popular Chinese dessert. Feel free to add more fruit, whatever is in season. If you have a hard time getting your children to eat healthy desserts, this will be a good start.

1¼ CUPS BREWED GREEN TEA (PAGE 39)

1 CUP GLUTINOUS RICE, ALSO CALLED SWEET RICE (PAGE 56)

½ CUP CHOPPED FRESH MANGO

¼ CUP GREEN CANDIED CHERRIES, HALVED OR QUARTERED

¼ CUP RAISINS

¼ CUP DRIED TART CHERRIES

¼ CUP CHOPPED CANDIED PINEAPPLE

½ CUP ALMOND BUTTER

¼ CUP MAPLE SYRUP

½ CUP GREEN TEA, MANGO, AND YOGURT SMOOTHIE,
    OPTIONAL (PAGE 286)

Place the green tea and rice in a rice cooker. Cook and set aside.

Line the bottom of a 6- to 8-inch bowl with plastic wrap. Artistically arrange the mango and the other fruit on the bottom of the bowl.

Pack half of the warm rice into the bowl in an even layer, following the curve of the bowl. Spread the almond butter and syrup on the rice.

Pack the remaining rice over the almond butter–syrup layer. Flatten the top of the rice firmly.

Place a platter on top of the bowl and invert, holding them together. Carefully lift off the bowl and remove the plastic wrap to reveal your fruit arrangement. Spoon the smoothie on top, if using. Serve warm.

Makes 4 servings

MORE USES FOR GREEN TEA

IN MANY ASIAN COUNTRIES, GREEN TEA IS USED FOR MEDICINAL AND OTHER PURPOSES. DO NOT DISCARD THE CONTENTS OF YOUR TEA BAGS, OR THE TEA LIQUID THAT'S LEFT OVER AFTER COOKING AND BREWING. THEY CAN BE USED FOR THE PURPOSES LISTED HERE.

+ FOR AN INFECTED TOOTH, PRESS ON BREWED TEA LEAVES TO STOP PAIN AND SWELLING.
+ FOR A FUNGAL FOOT INFECTION, BATHE THE FOOT IN STRONG BREWED TEA FOR 10 MINUTES TWICE A DAY FOR SEVERAL WEEKS.
+ FOR FRESH BREATH, CHEW BREWED TEA LEAVES.
+ RINSE YOUR MOUTH WITH STRONG TEA FOR CLEANING.
+ SPREAD BREWED TEA LEAVES AROUND THE ROOTS OF GARDEN PLANTS, ESPECIALLY ROSES AND PEPPERS. WITH USED TEA BAGS, TEAR OPEN THE BAG AND USE THE TEA. BREWED TEA LEAVES CONTAIN ORGANIC MATTER, WHICH MAKES A GOOD FERTILIZER FOR PLANTS.
+ ADD BREWED TEA AND LEFTOVER LIQUID TEA TO YOUR COMPOST PILE.
+ BURN DRY TEA LEAVES IN A POT TO DRIVE MOSQUITOES AWAY.

New Year's Rice Cake

Just as my son anxiously awaits his Christmas gifts for months in advance, as a child I anxiously awaited my New Year's Rice Cake. And like my son, your children will enjoy helping you prepare this simple, yummy delight.

1 POUND GLUTINOUS RICE FLOUR, ALSO CALLED
    SWEET RICE FLOUR (PAGE 57)

1 ¼ CUPS SUGAR

1 TABLESPOON BAKING POWDER

¼ CUP DRIED CHERRIES

¼ CUP CHOPPED CANDIED PINEAPPLE

¼ CUP DRIED DATES

¼ CUP CHOPPED NUTS

3 EGGS

¾ CUP CANOLA OIL

1 ½ CUPS WATER

RAISINS, NUTS, AND DRIED CHERRIES, FOR DECORATION

Preheat the oven to 375°F (175°C). Coat a 9-inch round cake pan with nonstick cooking spray.

Combine the rice flour, sugar, baking powder, cherries, pineapple, dates, and nuts in a large mixing bowl. Mix thoroughly. In a separate bowl, beat the eggs. Add the oil and water to the eggs and stir to combine.

Pour the egg mixture into the fruit mixture. Mix well. Pour the batter into the prepared pan.

Bake for 40 minutes, or until a knife inserted into the center comes out clean. The cake will rise when done.

Decorate the cake with three raisins each for eyes, nuts for the nose, and cherries for a smiling mouth.

Makes 8 servings

Asian Pears in Ginseng Sauce

Asian pears are also called Chinese or apple pears. They have a rounder shape and more juice than American pears. When I was small and had a cough, Grandmother would steam Asian pears with ginger and rock sugar. Chinese doctors believe this cooling combination soothes the lungs and throat and helps cure dry coughs.

Once steamed, the pears absorb the sweet sugar and become very tender. If you don't have rock sugar, use honey instead.

4 RIPE ASIAN PEARS OR OTHER FRESH PEARS

4 QUARTER-SIZE SLICES GINGER, LIGHTLY CRUSHED

4 TABLESPOONS ROCK SUGAR, BROKEN INTO SMALL PIECES (PAGE 57)

GLAZED CHERRIES, TO DECORATE

Peel the pears. With a melon baller, remove the core and seeds. Remove the stems. Do not cut through the bottoms of the pears.

Stuff 1 piece of ginger and 1 tablespoon rock sugar inside each pear. Arrange pears upright in a heatproof bowl.

Fill a wok or a vegetable steamer with water. Set the bowl on a steam rack. Bring water to a boil. Steam the pears until they are tender and the rock sugar has melted, 15 to 20 minutes.

Decorate each pear with cherries. Serve hot.

Makes 4 servings

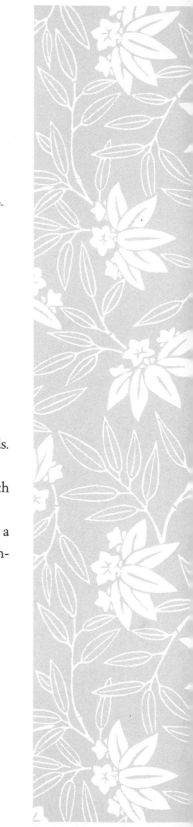

ASIAN BEAUTY SECRETS

GINSENG

Chinese emperors were famous for having hundreds of concubines. To maintain their beauty and pass the time, the concubines used the best ginseng root to brew soup for washing their hair and for their baths. I have found modern, simple ways to add ginseng to your beauty regimen.

For your hair: You will need 2 tablespoons of Asian ginseng powder, or you can grind ginseng tea in a grinder. Mix with a bottle of hair conditioner. Let the conditioner stay on your hair an extra 3 to 4 minutes. For the best results, after applying ginseng conditioner wrap your hair in a moist towel, put on a shower cap, set your blow dryer to low, and give your hair a heat treatment. You will be surprised at how good your hair will feel and look.

For your skin: Beautiful concubines in China were famous for taking baths with rose petals and herbs to get smooth, soft skin. Save the ginseng teabags after you brew the tea. When you take a hot bath, throw in 3 or 4 teabags. Add some rose petals or a couple of drops of rose oil. This will leave your skin feeling refreshed and smooth.

For beautiful plants: I have found that my houseplants love ginseng, too. Give them your leftover tea and used teabags. Open the teabags and spread the ginseng around the roots. Discard the bags.

Peanut Butter–Raisin Cookies

Before Christmas, I developed this recipe. My son helped me make the cookies and wrap them. We gave them to friends for Christmas. They were a big hit.

½ CUP LOW-FAT BUTTER OR MARGARINE

¼ CUP SUGAR

½ CUP CREAMY PEANUT BUTTER

1 EGG, LIGHTLY BEATEN

1 TEASPOON VANILLA EXTRACT

¾ CUP ALL-PURPOSE FLOUR

1 TABLESPOON POWDERED GINGER

½ TEASPOON BAKING SODA

¼ CUP RAISINS

Preheat the oven to 350°F (175°C). To a large heatproof bowl, add the butter and sugar. Place in the heated oven for 3 to 5 minutes, or until the butter starts to soften. Beat in the peanut butter, egg, and vanilla until light and fluffy.

In a medium bowl, combine the flour, ginger, and baking soda. Blend into creamed mixture. Stir in the raisins.

Spray a 1-tablespoon measuring spoon with cooking spray. Spoon balls of dough onto cookie sheets, about 2 inches apart.

Bake for 13 to 15 minutes, or until cookies are lightly browned. Let cookies cool completely. Store in an airtight container.

Makes 25 to 30 cookies

TIPS

PLACING THE BUTTER AND SUGAR IN THE HEATED OVEN, WHICH HELPS SOFTEN THE BUTTER, MAKES IT EASIER TO MIX. YOU CAN ALSO BRING THE BUTTER TO ROOM TEMPERATURE IN YOUR KITCHEN BEFORE USING.

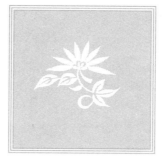

Soy-Chocolate Fantasy

Staying healthy does not mean you have to give up your passion for chocolate. Here is another recipe where East meets West.

1 (12.5-OUNCE) PACKAGE SOFT SILKEN TOFU

½ CUP HONEY

1 LARGE PARTIALLY FROZEN BANANA

1 TEASPOON VANILLA EXTRACT

¼ CUP SEMISWEET DARK CHOCOLATE CHIPS

¼ CUP SLICED ALMONDS, TOASTED

In a blender blend the tofu, honey, banana, and vanilla at high speed until smooth. Fold in the chocolate chips. Pour into serving glasses. Cover and refrigerate for 1 hour. Decorate with the almond slices.

Makes 4 servings

Pistachio Ice Cream

Believe it or not, you don't need an ice-cream maker to make ice cream. My family in China didn't own a refrigerator until I was in high school. That summer, my brothers and I tried to freeze all kinds of things. Making ice cream in the freezer was one of our greatest discoveries. The combination of ginger and pistachio is as unusual as it is irresistible.

2 CUPS LOW-FAT MILK

1½ TABLESPOONS SLICED GINGER

½ CUP SUGAR

1 SMALL RIPE BANANA

1 CUP WHIPPED TOPPING

½ CUP FINELY CHOPPED PISTACHIO NUTS
    PLUS 2 TABLESPOONS, FOR GARNISH

Combine the milk and ginger slices in a saucepan. Bring to a boil. Reduce heat to low and stir. Simmer for 5 minutes. Add the sugar, and cook, stirring, until sugar is dissolved.

Let cool. Remove and discard the ginger slices. Pour the mixture into a blender, and add the banana. Blend until smooth, 2 to 3 minutes.

Pour into a large bowl; gently fold in the whipped topping and ½ cup nuts. Pour the mixture into 4 small (about 1-cup) baking dishes or custard cups. Cover and freeze overnight.

Before serving, dip the outside of the dishes in cold water for 2 to 3 minutes. Holding a small plate over each dish, flip over, and unmold the ice cream. Decorate with remaining pistachio nuts.

Makes 4 servings

Banana-Soy Ice Cream

After a friend showed me how she makes ice cream with her ice-cream maker, I started to research ice-cream makers on the market (see pages 43–44 for more information) and found some wonderful models.

The garlic in this recipe heightens the taste of the banana in a new and delightful way.

2 CUPS SOYMILK

¼ TEASPOON MINCED GARLIC

½ CUP SUGAR

1 SMALL RIPE BANANA

¼ CUP FINELY CHOPPED PECANS PLUS
    2 TABLESPOONS, FOR GARNISH

Place the soymilk and garlic in a saucepan. Bring to a boil. Reduce heat to low and stir. Simmer for 5 minutes. Add the sugar, and cook, stirring, until sugar is dissolved.

Let cool. Pour the mixture into a blender and add the banana and pecans. Blend until smooth, 2 to 3 minutes.

Pour the mixture into an ice-cream maker. Freeze according to the ice-cream maker's instructions.

Scoop the ice cream into serving dishes. Decorate with remaining pecans before serving.

Makes 4 servings

Watermelon Sorbet

Watermelon is cooling, or yin. This is a great summertime treat after hot outdoor activities.

2 CUPS DICED, SEEDED WATERMELON

1 CUP VANILLA SOYMILK

1 CUP SOY CREAMER OR HEAVY CREAM

½ CUP SUGAR

MINT LEAVES, FOR GARNISH

Place all the ingredients, except mint, in a blender, and blend until smooth, about 2 minutes.

Pour the mixture into an ice-cream maker. Freeze according to the ice-cream maker's instructions.

Scoop the ice cream into serving dishes. Decorate with mint leaves.

Makes 4 to 6 servings

Black-Sesame Ice Cream

The first time I tasted black-sesame ice cream I was in the Tokyo airport. It was the best ice cream I ever had. After I got home, this was the first recipe I tested. I am so delighted to find another way to enjoy black sesame. Chinese women believe that eating black sesame keeps their hair lustrous and prevents it from turning gray.

1 CUP VANILLA SOYMILK

2 CUPS SOY CREAMER OR HEAVY CREAM

1 CUP CREAMED HAZELNUT HONEY (AVAILABLE IN
    HEALTH-FOOD STORES) OR REGULAR HONEY

1 CUP BLACK SESAME SEEDS, TOASTED
    (SEE PAGE 200)

CHERRIES, TO DECORATE

Place all the ingredients, except cherries, in a blender, and blend until smooth, about 2 minutes.

Pour the mixture into an ice-cream maker. Freeze according to the ice-cream maker's instructions.

Scoop the ice cream into serving dishes. Decorate with cherries.

Makes 6 servings

Ginger-Peach Ice Cream

Ginger and peach are a delicious combination. The cooling ice cream and peach are balanced by the fiery ginger.

2 (16-OUNCE) CANS PEACHES

2 TEASPOONS POWDERED GINGER

1½ CUPS SOY CREAMER OR HEAVY CREAM

½ CUP SUGAR

Place all the ingredients in a blender or food processor and blend until smooth, about 3 minutes.

Pour the mixture into an ice-cream maker. Freeze according to the ice-cream maker's instructions.

Scoop the ice cream into serving dishes.

Makes 6 servings

Green Tea Ice Cream

Here's another example of how "bland" tofu is more than just a health-conscious foodstuff. The kiwifruit adds a touch of green to the ice cream, but you can substitute other fruit.

Being a vegetarian doesn't mean you have to bypass ice cream. Traditionally, ice cream requires cow's milk and cream. I have experimented a bit and found that with soymilk and soy whipped topping, it comes out just as delicious.

1 CUP PLAIN OR VANILLA SOYMILK

4 GREEN TEA BAGS

1 (12-OUNCE) PACKAGE LOW-FAT FIRM SILKEN TOFU

½ CUP CREAMED HAZELNUT HONEY OR REGULAR HONEY

1 TABLESPOON VANILLA EXTRACT

2 KIWIFRUIT, PEELED AND DICED INTO CHUNKS

1 CUP SOY WHIPPED TOPPING

2 OR 3 DROPS GREEN FOOD COLORING (OPTIONAL)

Place the soymilk and teabags in a medium saucepan. Bring to a boil, reduce heat, and simmer for 5 minutes. Stir frequently to prevent scorching. Remove from heat and let cool.

Use two spoons to gently squeeze absorbed milk out of tea bags and discard the tea bags.

In a blender, combine the tofu, green tea milk, honey, vanilla, and kiwifruit. Blend until mixture is smooth, 2 to 3 minutes.

Pour blended mixture into a bowl suitable for freezing. Gently fold the whipped topping into the blended mixture. Cover and freeze for 5 to 6 hours, or until firm.

Makes 4 to 6 servings

TIPS

AN EASY WAY TO MEASURE THE HONEY IS TO FIRST TRANSFER THE GREEN TEA-MILK INTO A LARGE LIQUID MEASURING CUP. ADD HONEY UNTIL THE VOLUME HAS INCREASED BY $\frac{1}{2}$ CUP. THE MILK WILL HELP KEEP THE HONEY FROM STICKING TO THE MEASURING CUP AS YOU POUR IT INTO THE BLENDER.

A FRIEND WHO TOOK A COOKING CLASS FROM A SUSHI CHEF TOLD ME THE SECRET FOR "MAKING" EASY GREEN TEA ICE CREAM. SOFTEN 1 CUP REGULAR VANILLA ICE CREAM, MIX WITH $\frac{1}{2}$ TEASPOON MACHA CEREMONY TEA, THEN RETURN THE ICE CREAM TO THE FREEZER. ONCE IT'S FIRM IT IS READY TO SERVE. BUT YOU CAN TELL YOUR FRIENDS IT WAS VERY COMPLICATED TO MAKE. YOU CAN ORDER MACHA TEA (SEE PAGE 298) OR BUY IT AT SOME ASIAN MARKETS.

Green Tea, Mango, and Yogurt Smoothie

A great way to start your day—the green tea wakes you up gently and the protein gives you lasting energy.

4 JASMINE GREEN TEA BAGS

1 CUP HOT WATER

2 LARGE MANGOES

12 ICE CUBES

2 TABLESPOONS HONEY

2 (6-OUNCE) CARTONS SOY APRICOT OR MANGO YOGURT

Brew tea bags in the hot water for 5 minutes to best extract the green tea flavor. Use two spoons to remove the tea bags and press out excess tea. Discard the tea bags and let the tea cool.

Peel, seed, and cube the mangoes.

Place the ice cubes in a blender and blend at medium speed for 10 seconds. Add the mangoes, green tea, honey, and yogurt. Blend at medium speed until smooth and frosty, about 15 seconds.

Serve immediately for best color and taste, or store in a tightly sealed container in refrigerator until serving time.

Makes 4 cups

Blueberry-Banana Shake

For the best color and flavor, serve immediately. The shake can be covered and refrigerated for one day.

1 (12.5-OUNCE) PACKAGE SOFT SILKEN TOFU

1½ CUPS FROZEN BLUEBERRIES

1 RIPE MEDIUM BANANA

1 TABLESPOON HONEY

4 STRAWBERRIES, TO DECORATE

Place all the ingredients, except the strawberries, in a blender and blend at high speed until smooth. Pour into glasses and decorate with the strawberries.

Makes 4 servings

Ginger, Mango, and Yogurt Smoothie

This luxurious fruit smoothie is one of my favorites. I often make it to reward myself after my morning workout. You can substitute peaches, berries, or papaya for the mango. You can also substitute a banana for the yogurt.

2 MEDIUM MANGOES

12 ICE CUBES

4 QUARTER-SIZE SLICES YOUNG GINGER

2 TABLESPOONS HONEY

1 CUP PINEAPPLE-COCONUT JUICE

2 (6-OUNCE) CARTONS MANGO AND APRICOT
    YOGURT OR OTHER FRUIT YOGURT

Peel, seed, and cube the mangoes.

Place the ice cubes, ginger, and honey in a blender and blend at medium speed for 10 seconds. Add the mangoes, juice, and yogurt. Blend at medium speed until smooth and frosty, about 30 seconds.

Serve immediately for best color and taste, or store in a tightly sealed container in the refrigerator until serving time.

Makes 4 1/2 cups

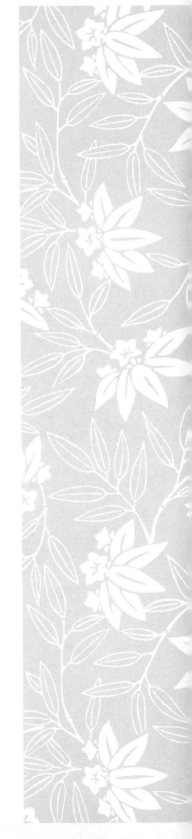

Sunrise Smoothie

A green tea–fruit smoothie I had at a beach resort in China was the inspiration for this recipe. Since then, it has become a favorite morning drink. Next time you need a caffeinated wake-up call, try this simple, tasty, and nutritious smoothie. Use the number of tea bags that suits your morning mood. An average cup (6 ounces) of green tea brewed with one tea bag contains about 30 milligrams of caffeine. Compare this to a cup of brewed coffee that has 120 milligrams of caffeine.

2 MEDIUM BANANAS, CUT INTO 1-INCH SLICES

4 KIWIFRUIT (ABOUT ¾ POUND), PEELED AND CUT INTO LARGE CUBES

4 FRUIT-FLAVORED GREEN TEA BAGS

1½ CUPS SOYMILK

1 TABLESPOON HONEY

CHERRIES, FOR GARNISH

Place the bananas and kiwifruit in a sealed plastic bag. Freeze for 30 minutes, or until almost firm.

Place the tea bags in a medium bowl. Bring the soymilk to a boil. Pour the soymilk over the tea bags; let the tea steep for 3 minutes. Remove the tea bags. Stir in the honey, and cool.

Combine the tea, banana, and kiwifruit in a blender. Blend at high speed until smooth, about 1 minute. Pour into glasses and top with cherries.

Makes 4 cups

TIP
TO SPEED UP THE RIPENING TIME OF BANANAS, PLACE A COUPLE OF ORANGES AROUND THEM. ORANGES GIVE OFF ETHYLENE GAS, WHICH ACCELERATES THE RIPENING OF THE BANANAS.

Midlife Boost

Research studies have shown that soy contains phytoestrogens that help women with menopause. For centuries, Chinese women have also recommended taking ginseng and dong quai *(see page 52) to relieve distressing menopausal symptoms.*

Serve this drink the next time you are having a women's party or after your yoga class. But if you are pregnant or lactating, talk to your Chinese doctor before using dong quai *and ginseng.*

1 (16-OUNCE) BOTTLE CHAI (A MIXTURE OF TEA, MILK, AND
    SPICES, AVAILABLE AT MOST HEALTH-FOOD STORES)

2 CUPS SOYMILK

4 PIECES OF FRESH OR DRY GINSENG SLICES

4 PIECES *DONG QUAI*

In a large heavy pot, mix the chai, soymilk, ginseng, and *dong quai*. Bring to a boil. Reduce heat and simmer for 25 to 30 minutes. Serve hot.

Makes 6 to 8 servings

VARIATION

IF YOU DON'T HAVE GINSENG SLICES, USE GINSENG TEA BAGS INSTEAD.

NEW MOTHERS AND *DONG QUAI*

I remember how surprised I was when one of my American friends told me she went back to work a week after having her baby. In China, new mothers stay indoors and avoid heavy housework for a whole month.

During this time the new mother is served a diet composed mainly of yang foods to replenish her energy and help produce milk. Chinese ginseng, *dong quai*, and dates have been used for centuries by Chinese women after their menstrual cycle, and after giving birth, to restore the harmony of hormones, and lost blood, to invigorate the reproductive system, improve circulation, maintain youth, and eliminate menopausal symptoms, such as hot flashes.

After my son was born, I received packages of ginseng, *dong quai*, and dates from my Chinese friends. (I was instructed to make the drink on page 292; take it for 30 days; and avoid wind, dampness, and cold foods, including cold water.)

Restoring Feminine Tonic

Historically, Chinese doctors have believed dong quai *(see page 52) replenishes blood supply and improves circulation. It is used to treat symptoms of low blood pressure—weakness and dizziness. It is also prescribed for irregular menstrual cycles and cramps as well as arthritis. In a recent study in China, surgeons attested to* dong quai's *ability to improve circulation in damaged tissues, using it in treating trauma to ease pain and reduce bruising.*

The dong quai *has a pronounced aroma when it is cooking, and a strong flavor. It is an acquired taste.*

4 PIECES FRESH OR DRY GINSENG ROOTS (ABOUT 2 OUNCES)

4 TO 6 PIECES *DONG QUAI* (ABOUT 3 OUNCES)

8 DRIED BLACK OR RED CHINESE DATES (PAGE 52)

6 CUPS COLD WATER

1 ½ OUNCES ROCK SUGAR (ABOUT 3 TABLESPOONS) (PAGE 57)

In a large saucepan, combine the ginseng, *dong quai*, dates, and cold water. Bring to a boil. Cover and reduce heat to medium-low, and simmer until the liquid is reduced to 4 cups, about 50 minutes.

Serve warm. Store the remainder in the refrigerator in a sealed glass jar and heat before serving.

Makes 4 servings

TIPS
I LIKE TO EAT THE GINSENG AND *DONG QUAI* AT THE END, BUT THEY HAVE A VERY STRONG FLAVOR.

YOU CAN FIND CHINESE DATES AT ASIAN MARKETS.

Summer Fruit Shake

This is a perfect after-dinner beverage. It goes especially well outdoors after a barbecue. The cooling effect of American ginseng and melon will balance the yang of grilled meat. It leaves you feeling fresh and cool.

2½ CUPS SPRING WATER

2 PIECES FRESH OR DRY AMERICAN GINSENG, SLICED

2 CUPS SEEDLESS WATERMELON CUBES

2 CUPS CANTALOUPE CUBES

1 CUP HONEYDEW CUBES

6 ICE CUBES

MINT LEAVES, FOR GARNISH

In a saucepan, bring the water to a boil. Add the ginseng slices. Reduce heat to low and simmer until reduced to about 2 cups, about 20 minutes. Let it cool.

Place the ginseng tea, including the ginseng slices, and all the fruit into a food processor or blender. Blend until fruit is pureed, 2 to 3 minutes.

Pour into glasses and garnish with mint leaves. Serve immediately for the best taste and color.

Makes 4 to 6 servings

Soy-Coconut Milk Shake

Next time you feel an urge for a healthy, delicious drink, give this one a try. It is very calming and nurturing for your digestive system. In general, coconut milk is high in fat but in this recipe I combined it with soymilk, which is lower in fat. You get the flavor of coconut and the health benefit of soy all in one.

½ (12-OUNCE) PACKAGE SOFT SILKEN TOFU

3 CUPS SOYMILK

1 CUP COCONUT MILK

3 TABLESPOONS HONEY

1 CUP ICE CUBES

2 TABLESPOONS PISTACHIO NUTS,
    SHELLED AND FINELY CHOPPED

In a blender, combine the tofu, soymilk, coconut milk, and honey and blend until frothy. Pour over ice. Garnish with pistachio nuts.

Makes 6 servings

Apple Cider

This is a wonderful drink for a cool day. It helps your body restore energy and recover from an illness.

1 PACKAGE HOT CIDER SPICES OR MULLING SPICES

2 CUPS FRESH APPLE JUICE

6 PIECES FRESH OR DRY ASIAN GINSENG SLICES OR TEA BAGS

Cut out two (8-inch) squares of cheesecloth. Layer them on top of each other. Place spices in the middle. Tie the corners together to form a bag. Place the apple juice, spice mixture, and ginseng in a big heavy pot. Bring to a boil. Reduce heat to low and simmer for 30 minutes. Serve hot.

Makes 8 to 10 servings

> **TIP**
>
> THIS DRINK KEEPS WELL IN THE REFRIGERATOR FOR 3 TO 4 DAYS. LET IT COOL PRIOR TO STORING IN A SEALED GLASS JAR. REHEAT ON THE STOVE OR IN THE MICROWAVE BEFORE SERVING.

Honeyed-Ginseng Sun Tea

This is a great summertime beverage. While the yin effect of American ginseng helps cool your body from the summer heat, the honey enhances your digestion system. The drink will last in the refrigerator for 3 to 4 days.

5 PIECES AMERICAN GINSENG SLICES,
    OR 4 GINSENG TEA BAGS

6 CUPS COLD WATER

HONEY TO TASTE

Place the ginseng and water in a glass jar. Set the jar in the hot summer sun for 3 to 5 hours.

Place the jar in the refrigerator. Serve with or without ice. Drizzle in a little honey before serving.

NOTE

TO MAKE THIS ON A CLOUDY DAY, BRING GINSENG OR TEA BAGS TO A BOIL AND LET IT SIMMER FOR 10 MINUTES. COOL AND STORE IN THE REFRIGERATOR.

OR STEEP THE GINSENG SLICES OR TEA BAGS IN HALF THE WATER (3 CUPS). POUR INTO A CONTAINER FILLED WITH ICE. THE ICE WILL SIMULTANEOUSLY DILUTE THE TEA AND CHILL IT.

Resources

During the course of researching this book, I tested many products and foods. I found those made by the following companies to be superior. I've listed the companies' websites and phone numbers for your convenience.

Cookware

Calphalon Corporation
www.calphalon.com
(800) 809-7262
nonstick wok, chef's pan, stove-top grill pan

Le Creuset of America, Inc.
www.lecreuset.com
(800) 827-1789
saucepan, French oven, and teakettle

Zojirushi American Corporation
www.zojirushi.com
(800) 733-6270
rice cooker, electric dispensing pot (hot water for tea and cooking)

Appliances

KitchenAid
www.kitchenaid.com
(800) 422-1230
Energy Star® Qualified top-freezer
refrigerator

Ducane
www.ducane.com
(800) 382-2637
5004SS Gas Grill
The Open-Flame rotisserie cooks
from behind. The design minimizes
flareups and there's no grease trap to
clean, plus there's the convenience
of two burners for grilling and one
side burner for sauté or stir-fry.

Donvier
www.donvier.com
Nonelectric Ice Cream Maker

Kitchen Knives

Zwilling J. A. Henckels, Inc.
www.j-a-henckels.com
Five Star and Twinstar Plus Knives

Organic Foods

Eden Foods, Inc.
www.edenfoods.com
(888) 424-3336
Soy sauces, tamari, rice vinegar,
sesame oil, flavored sesame shakes,
extra virgin olive oil, udon and soba
noodles, soymilk, toasted nori, and a
variety of other pasta and Asian
ingredients.

GINSENG
HSU's Ginseng Enterprises, Inc.
www.hsuginseng.com
(800) 826-1577
Fresh and dry ginseng root, whole, in
slices and in teabags.

Teas and Teapots

Celestial Seasonings
www.celestialseasonings.com
(800) 697-7887
Bagged green teas, ginseng tea, and
yixing teapots.

Water and Leaves Company
www.wayoftea.com
(800) 699-4753
Loose tea and yixing teapots

Conversion Tables

Comparison to Metric Measure

When You Know	Symbol	Multiply By	To Find	Symbol
teaspoons	tsp.	5.0	milliliters	ml
tablespoons	tbsp.	15.0	milliliters	ml
fluid ounces	fl. oz.	30.0	milliliters	ml
cups	c	0.24	liters	l
pints	pt.	0.47	liters	l
quarts	qt.	0.95	liters	l
ounces	oz.	28.0	grams	g
pounds	lb.	0.45	kilograms	kg
Fahrenheit	F	5/9 (after subtracting 32)	Celsius	C

Liquid Measure to Milliliters

$\frac{1}{4}$	teaspoon	=	1.25	milliliters
$\frac{1}{2}$	teaspoon	=	2.5	milliliters
$\frac{3}{4}$	teaspoon	=	3.75	milliliters
1	teaspoon	=	5.0	milliliters
$1\frac{1}{4}$	teaspoons	=	6.25	milliliters
$1\frac{1}{2}$	teaspoons	=	7.5	milliliters
$1\frac{3}{4}$	teaspoons	=	8.75	milliliters
2	teaspoons	=	10.0	milliliters
1	tablespoon	=	15.0	milliliters
2	tablespoons	=	30.0	milliliters

Fahrenheit to Celsius

F	C
200–205	95
220–225	105
245–250	120
275	135
300–305	150
325–330	165
345–350	175
370–375	190
400–405	205
425–430	220
445–450	230
470–475	245
500	260

Liquid Measure to Liters

¼	cup	=	0.06	liters
½	cup	=	0.12	liters
¾	cup	=	0.18	liters
1	cup	=	0.24	liters
1¼	cups	=	0.3	liters
1½	cups	=	0.36	liters
2	cups	=	0.48	liters
2½	cups	=	0.6	liters
3	cups	=	0.72	liters
3½	cups	=	0.84	liters
4	cups	=	0.96	liters
4½	cups	=	1.08	liters
5	cups	=	1.2	liters
5½	cups	=	1.32	liters

Index

ABOUT THE AUTHOR

Ying Chang Compestine was born and raised in China. After relocating to the United States in 1986, she earned her master's degree from the University of Colorado.

Ying has a longtime passion for food and cultural diversity. Blended with her interest in health, this has inspired her writings on healthy Asian cooking. In addition, she has written a series of children's books that emphasize Chinese food and culture.

Ying and her healthy Asian cuisine have been featured on numerous television and radio shows. She has been profiled in magazines and newspapers across the country. She appears regularly on the Discovery Channel's *Home Matters*.

Ying has taught classes in healthy Asian cooking throughout the United States and speaks about healthy eating and living on renowned cruise lines around the world.

Ying is also a regular contributor to national magazines such as *Cooking Light* and *Delicious Living*.

She lives in Colorado with her husband and son.